The History of Medicine

Renaissance Medicine

Ian Dawson

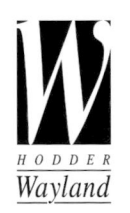

Wayland

HODDER

an imprint of Hodder Children's Books

First published in 2005 by Hodder Wayland,
an imprint of Hodder Children's Books

© Hodder Wayland 2005

Commissioning editor: Victoria Brooker
Editor: Deborah Fox
Inside design: Peta Morey
Cover design: Hodder Wayland
Picture research: Shelley Noronha, Glass Onion Pictures
Consultant: Dr Peter Elmer, Senior Lecturer, Dept of the History of Science,
Technology and Medicine, The Open University

British Library Cataloguing in Publication Data:

Dawson, Ian, 1951 Aug. 25-
The Renaissance. - (History of medicine)
1.Medicine - Europe - History - 16th century - Juvenile literature
2.Medicine - Europe - History - 15th century - Juvenile literature
I.Title
610.9'4'09031

ISBN 0 7502 4641 3

Printed and bound in China

Hodder Children's Books
A division of Hodder Headline Limited
338 Euston Road, London NW1 3BH

The author and publisher would like to thank the following for allowing their
pictures to be reproduced in this publication: AKG Images 7, 11, 17, 33, 35, 41,
45, AKG Images/Erich Lessing 6; The Art Archive/Dagli Orti (A) 4, The Art
Archive/Biblioteca Nacional Madrid/Dagli Orti 10, The Art Archive/Musée des Beaux
Arts Orléans/Dagli Orti (A) 25, The Art Archive, Museo del Prado Madrid 26, The Art
Archive/Dagli Orti 28, The Art Archive/Palazzo del Te Mantua/Dagli Orti (A) 29, The
Art Archive/Mireille Vautier 32, The Art Archive/Museo del Prado Madrid 39, The Art
Archive/Collection de la Faculté de Medicine Paris/Marc Charmet 43, The Art
Archive/Correr Venice/Dagli Orti (A) 1, 49, The Art Archive 50, The Art
Archive/Private Collection/Eileen Tweedy 55; Bridgeman Art Library 18, 54,
Bridgeman Art Library/Archives Charmet 8, 9, 15, 42, Bridgeman/Lauros/Giraudon
12, Bridgeman Art Library/Alinari 13, Bridgeman Art Library/Giraudon 16, 48, 59,
Royal College of Physicians London/Bridgeman Art Library 19, The Wellington
Museum London/Bridgeman Art Library 24, Ken Walsh/Bridgeman Art Library 27, The
Stapleton Collection/Bridgeman Art Library 31, Royal Society of Arts/Bridgeman Art
Library 38, Cheltenham Art Gallery & Museums, Gloucestershire/Bridgeman Art
Library 40, Johnny van Haeften Gallery, London/Bridgeman Art Library 46, Private
Collection/Bridgeman Art Library 51, 52, 53, Glasgow University Library,
Scotland/Bridgeman Art Library 57; © Michael Nicholson/CORBIS 34; Topham 5, 61;
Wellcome Library, London 3, 14, 21, 22, 23, 30, 36 and cover, 37, 44, 47, 56

Contents

Chapter 1

The world of the Renaissance

The period from 1450 to 1750, which began with the Renaissance of the fifteenth and sixteenth centuries, was a time of major medical discoveries. Doctors developed new approaches to the study of anatomy and so acquired more detailed and accurate knowledge of the structure of the human body. There were significant breakthroughs in the understanding of physiology (the workings of the human body), for example the discovery that the heart pumps the blood around the body. These and other breakthroughs were aided by technical and scientific inventions, such as the first microscopes.

The period of the fifteenth and sixteenth centuries, in particular, is often known as the Renaissance, which means 'rebirth', particularly the rebirth of the study of Greek and Roman knowledge and skills. During the

Artists and architects of the Renaissance period copied Ancient Greek and Roman styles. The façade of the Porta de Palio in Verona, designed by Sammicheli in 1561, includes columns that are similar to those in Greek temples and other buildings.

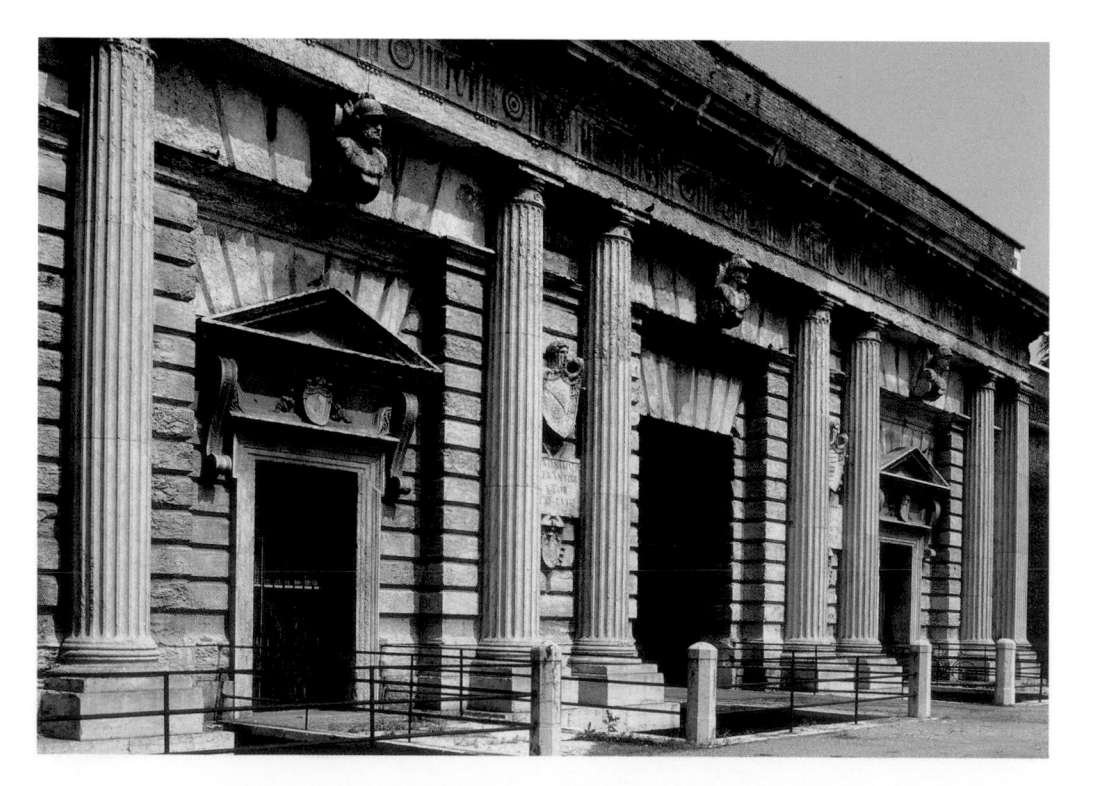

Renaissance, artists and scholars were rediscovering the glories of ancient architecture and learning and then asking questions about Greek and Roman ideas and challenging their traditions. Renaissance scholars, artists and scientists were therefore able to improve on ancient ideas and techniques. No one exemplified this passion for discovery and excellence more than Leonardo da Vinci.

This book, however, moves beyond the Renaissance of the fifteenth and sixteenth centuries to explore the continuing medical developments of the period up until the mid-eighteenth century. This is because the story of medical change at this time is one of slow development, with the discoveries of the sixteenth century gradually leading to further new ideas over the next two centuries. However, by the end of the eighteenth century, the work of doctors and scientists had finally overturned many of the traditional medical beliefs that had held sway since Greek and Roman times. The doctors and scientists had also established a foundation of knowledge that provided the launch pad for the astounding revolution in medicine and health that took place in the nineteenth and twentieth centuries.

The microscope was the most important medical instrument developed in this period, helping scientists to discover, for example, the existence of the capillaries, which transfer blood from the arteries to the veins. You can read more about the development and role of microscopes on page 21.

Renaissance Man – Leonardo da Vinci (1452–1519)

The man whose work most clearly exemplifies the vitality of the Renaissance was Leonardo da Vinci. Born in the small town of Vinci in Italy, he trained as an artist in the city of Florence and became famous for the delicacy and character of his paintings and drawings. However, da Vinci also worked as an engineer, designing canals, bridges and weapons and experimenting with ideas for submarines and flying machines. He studied all branches of science, including chemistry, astronomy and botany and he dissected human bodies in order to draw detailed illustrations of human anatomy, which made an important contribution to the development of medical understanding.

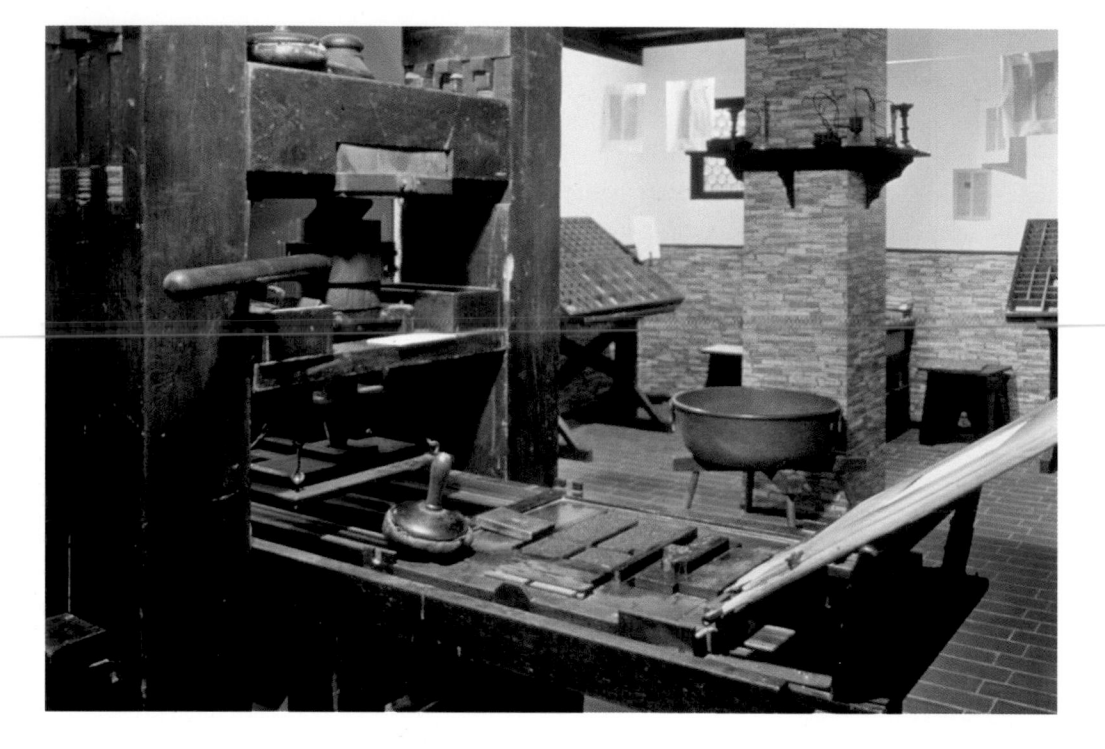

New ideas

Medical discoveries were part of the pattern of developments in the wider world of science. During the Renaissance many aspects of the world were being questioned and re-evaluated. The Polish mathematician Copernicus and the Italian astronomer Galileo proved that the earth rotates around the sun, rather than vice-versa. Isaac Newton, in the seventeenth century, established the law of gravity. Practical scientific developments also affected medicine. Clocks, watches and water-pumps were improved and the techniques used were applied to developing medical instruments, notably the earliest microscopes.

The influence of printing

However, the most important invention for the growth of medical knowledge was the printing press. It was invented in the mid-fifteenth century when the number of people who could read was rising rapidly, especially in the cities of Europe. Around half of fifteenth-century Londoners, for example, were literate.

A modern reproduction of the first printing press. Printing was developed in the mid-fifteenth century in Germany by Johannes Gutenberg and brought to England in the 1470s by William Caxton. Printing techniques meant that it was possible to reproduce a drawing many times and so it became possible to include accurate drawings in medical books.

Printing revolutionized communications. In the Middle Ages new ideas spread extremely slowly because all books and manuscripts were hand-written, which meant that it was almost impossible to create multiple copies of a text quickly. In addition, the Christian Church (which controlled education) had not encouraged scholars to pursue new ideas or to experiment. However, from the mid-fifteenth century onwards, the printing presses rapidly churned out hundreds or thousands of copies of books and so the ideas within them spread around Europe much more rapidly. Even the power of the Church could not stop the spread of ideas.

Among the first medical texts to be printed were those written by the Roman doctor, Galen. Galen's work had dominated medical studies throughout the Middle Ages and the development of printing meant that the scholars and students in universities could all have cheap printed editions of his works; few before could afford to buy their own copies of expensive hand-written manuscripts.

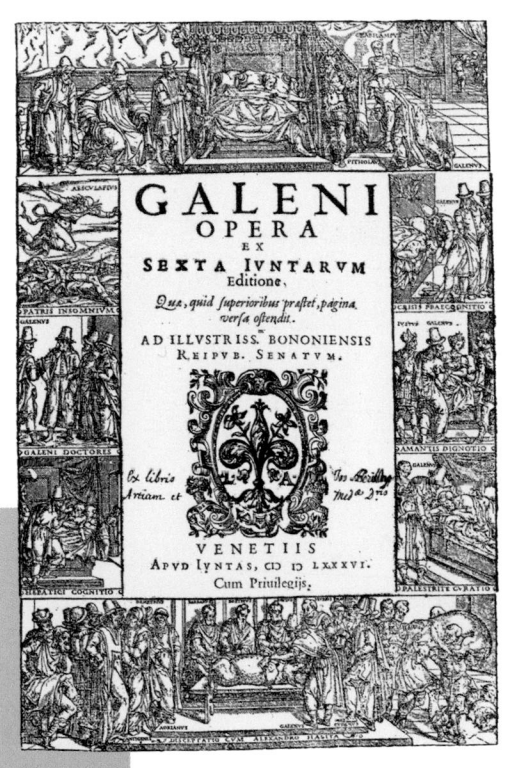

The title page of a collection of Galen's writings on medicine, published in Venice in 1586. The page shows scenes from Galen's life.

Galen, the 'Prince of Physicians'

The greatest names in medicine were the Greek 'Father of Medicine', Hippocrates (born c. 460 BCE) and the Roman, Claudius Galen (c. 130–200 CE). Galen built on the work of Hippocrates and other Greek doctors, adding his own theories developed from his own medical experience and from dissections of the bodies of both humans and animals. Galen wrote over 60 books, which remained the bedrock of medical training throughout the Middle Ages. Few doctors dared to challenge Galen's ideas, partly because his work was so detailed and convincing and partly because they had been trained to accept, rather than challenge, traditional beliefs.

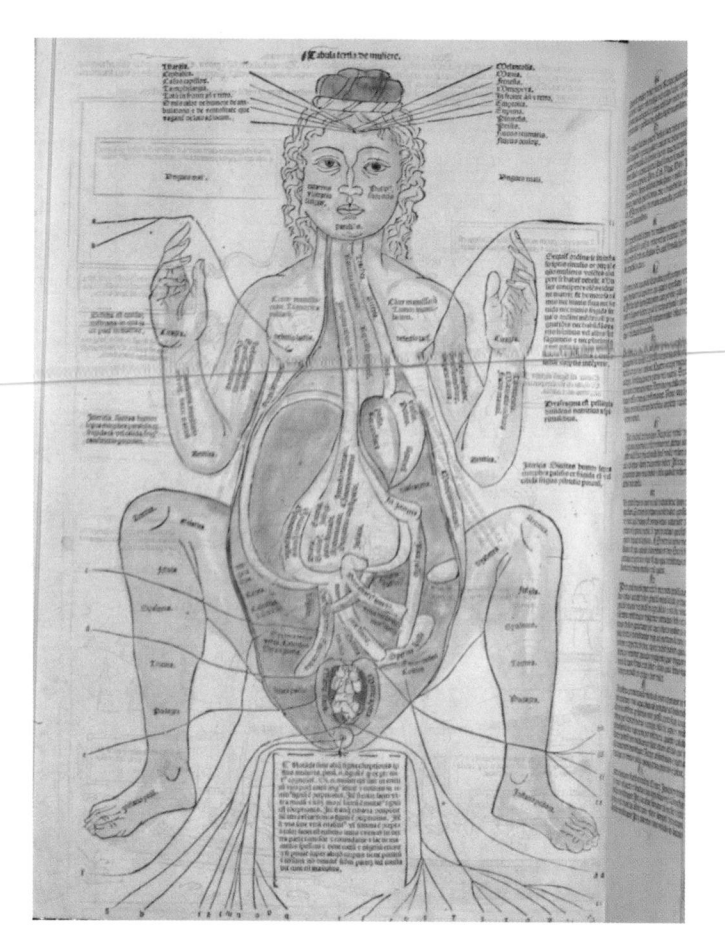

Medieval drawings look extremely simple, such as this late fifteenth-century Italian illustration of the anatomy of a pregnant woman, and we can fall into the trap of believing that medieval artists could not draw well, especially when compared to da Vinci's illustration opposite. However, medieval illustrators of the body did not aim to be realistic. They simply wanted to show main features.

The theory of the Four Humours

During the fourteenth and fifteenth centuries, as Renaissance ideas were developing, doctors were trained at university medical schools. The most respected were at Salerno, Padua and Bologna in Italy and at Paris and Montpellier in France. Students travelled from across Europe to train at these schools, where they read Galen's writings, along with the works of Hippocrates, other Greek and Roman writers and translations of Arab scholars such as Ibn Sina and al-Razi.

At the heart of the medical books was the theory of the Four Humours, which explained why people became ill. It had originated 3000 years earlier with Hippocrates and his followers and had been developed by Galen. The theory said that illnesses were caused when the

Four Humours, or liquids, in the body (blood, phlegm, black bile and yellow bile) fell out of balance. Therefore doctors tried to make the sick well by restoring the balance of the humours. This was usually done by bleeding or purging the patient to reduce the quantity of the humour believed to be overpowering the other humours.

"You will need three dissections!"

The following extracts from Leonard da Vinci's *Notebook*, 1519, give advice to young artists:

The painter who has a knowledge of sinews, muscles and tendons will know exactly which sinew causes the movement of a limb ... he will be able to show the various muscles in the different attitudes of his figures ... You will need three dissections to have a complete knowledge of the arteries, three more for the membranes, three for the nerves, muscles and ligaments, three for the bones and cartilages. Three must also be devoted to the female body ...

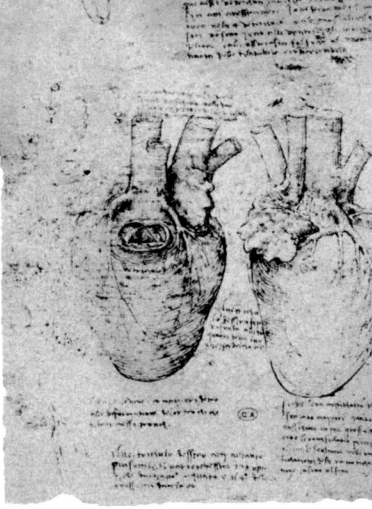

Art and medicine

During the Renaissance, the renewed interest in Greek and Roman ideas led scholars to seek out the original texts by Galen, to check translations and to see whether there was even more they could learn from the greatest of all doctors. Printed editions of these texts, in Greek and Latin, spread rapidly around Europe in the sixteenth century.

A particular attraction of these books was that many of them were well illustrated. Artists such as da Vinci believed that they had to study nature carefully in order to produce the most lifelike paintings and sculptures. Therefore, as you can read in the panel, da Vinci advised artists to carry out dissections to improve their knowledge of the human body. The results helped to revolutionize anatomical knowledge and the illustration of medical texts.

An anatomical illustration of the heart by Leonardo da Vinci. Unlike the medieval illustrators, da Vinci was striving for lifelike accuracy.

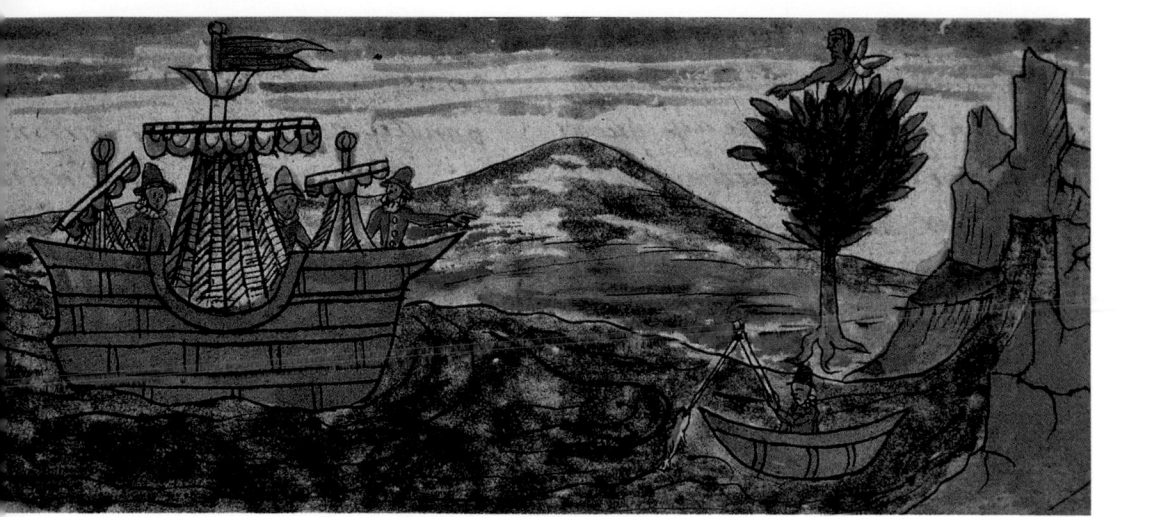

Exploration and the spread of disease

The Renaissance was an age of confidence and enquiry, but not all its effects were positive. The period saw the beginning of European exploration of the world, motivated by a desire for wealth, scientific knowledge and a wish to convert other peoples to Christianity from their own religions. However, wherever Europeans travelled, they took diseases with them.

In 1492 Columbus landed on the island of Hispaniola in the West Indies. Within a year, nearly half of the Arawak people of the island had died from influenza, carried by Columbus's men from Europe. The people of the Americas had not suffered from smallpox, measles, typhoid and scarlet fever and so had no immunity to them. The diseases killed millions.

A drawing from the *Historia de las Indias* by Diego Duran (1579), showing a native on the Mexican coast watching the arrival of Spanish ships. Voyages of exploration were made possible by improvements in the construction of ships and by the development of the compass and the astrolabe and quadrant, used for navigational purposes at sea.

Disease and the fall of civilizations

In 1521, the Spanish adventurer Hernan Cortes and 300 soldiers attacked the Aztec capital, Tenochtitlan (present-day Mexico City), home to 300,000 people. It should have been an impossible task, but the Aztecs were dying from smallpox, caught from earlier contacts with the invaders. When Cortes entered the city, he discovered that half the inhabitants had died and many others were ill. A decade later, it was smallpox, not guns and gunpowder, which enabled another Spaniard,

Pizarro, to capture the Incan city of Cuzco in modern Peru. Between 1518 and 1531, smallpox killed a third of the Aztec and Incan peoples and destroyed their great civilizations.

Diseases from Africa

The death toll in South and Central America created a problem for the Spanish, who needed workers for their silver-mines and farms. Their solution was to import slaves from Africa, who brought more new diseases, such as malaria and yellow fever. The diseases hit the surviving native peoples hard and also killed European immigrants to America. Yellow fever also made military service in the West Indies a death sentence for European troops. For example, in 1655 France sent 1500 men to invade the island of St Lucia in the West Indies. All but 89 died of the disease.

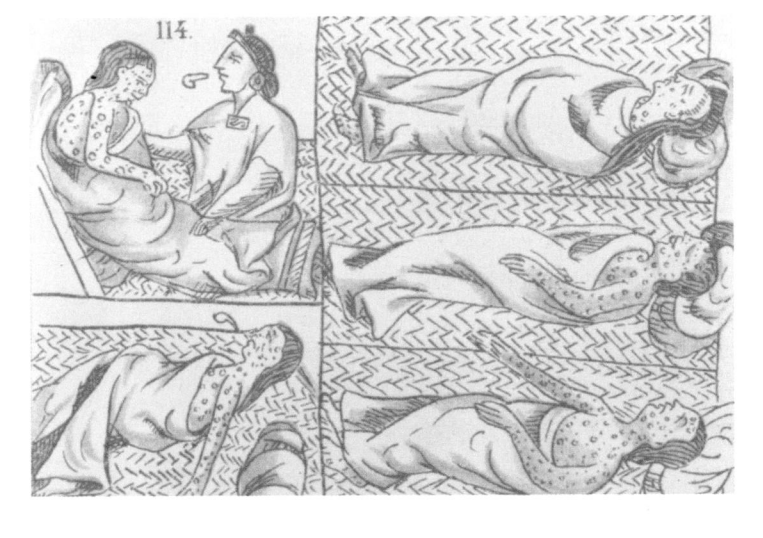

Drawings from an account of the Spanish conquest of Mexico by a missionary, Bernhardino de Span, c. 1570, showing local people ill with smallpox.

Smallpox hits North America

Diseases such as smallpox also hit the native peoples of North America, sometimes caught from infected blankets and clothes traded with European immigrants. In the mid-seventeenth century, for example, half of the Huron and Cherokee peoples died from smallpox. In the English colony of Massachusetts, the governor, John Winthrop, wrote in 1634, "God's hand hath so pursued the natives as, for three hundred miles space, the greatest part of them are swept away by the smallpox, which still continues amongst them. So, God hath hereby cleared our title to this space ...".

Chapter 2

Great medical discoveries

Vesalius and anatomy

One of the key figures of the medical world was Andreas Vesalius who became Professor of Surgery and Anatomy at the University of Padua when he was only 23. At Padua, Vesalius carried out many detailed dissections, usually of executed criminals, and this work was the basis for his great book *The Fabric of the Human Body*, published in 1543. This book revolutionized the way anatomical dissections were carried out and taught and it also showed that careful dissection could lead to new understandings of the structure of the human body.

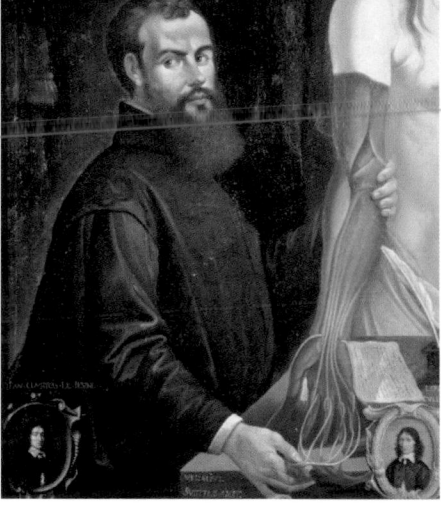

A portrait of Andreas Vesalius, 1514–1564, painted by Pierre Poncet. Vesalius was born in Brussels and his real name was van Wesele (Vesalius was the Latin version). His father was Royal Pharmacist to Emperor Charles V, providing enough money to help him begin his university education.

Until the fourteenth century, human dissection had not played any part in medical education. However, in the early 1300s, students at the university at Bologna in Italy were the first to be required to attend the dissection of a corpse as part of their studies. Then human dissections became an important, if small, part of medical education in Italy and Spain, although the students did not dissect the bodies themselves. They simply watched from the tiered

Stealing a body!

As a young man in Louvain, in present-day Belgium, Vesalius found a body to dissect on the gibbet outside the town, where the bodies of executed criminals were hanging. Later he told how:

The bones were entirely bare, held together by the ligaments alone ... I climbed the gallows and pulled off the femur from the hip bone ... after I had brought the legs and arms home in secret (leaving the head behind with the trunk of the body), I let myself be locked out of the city in the evening in order to obtain the trunk ... the next day I transported the bones home piecemeal.

seats in the newly built anatomy theatres while three people took part in the dissection. The professor, a qualified physician, was in charge; his assistant, the 'ostensor', pointed out the parts of the body and the lowliest member of the trio, the surgeon, did the actual dissection. This meant that the professor did not do the dissection himself and so was much less likely to be aware of any differences between the structure of the body and what was described in Galen's books.

Vesalius changed this approach, emphasizing that the professor should perform all three roles and so undertake detailed dissections himself. He knew from his own experience that new anatomical knowledge could only come from dissecting human bodies, rather than by dissecting animals or simply reading the books of Galen and other authors.

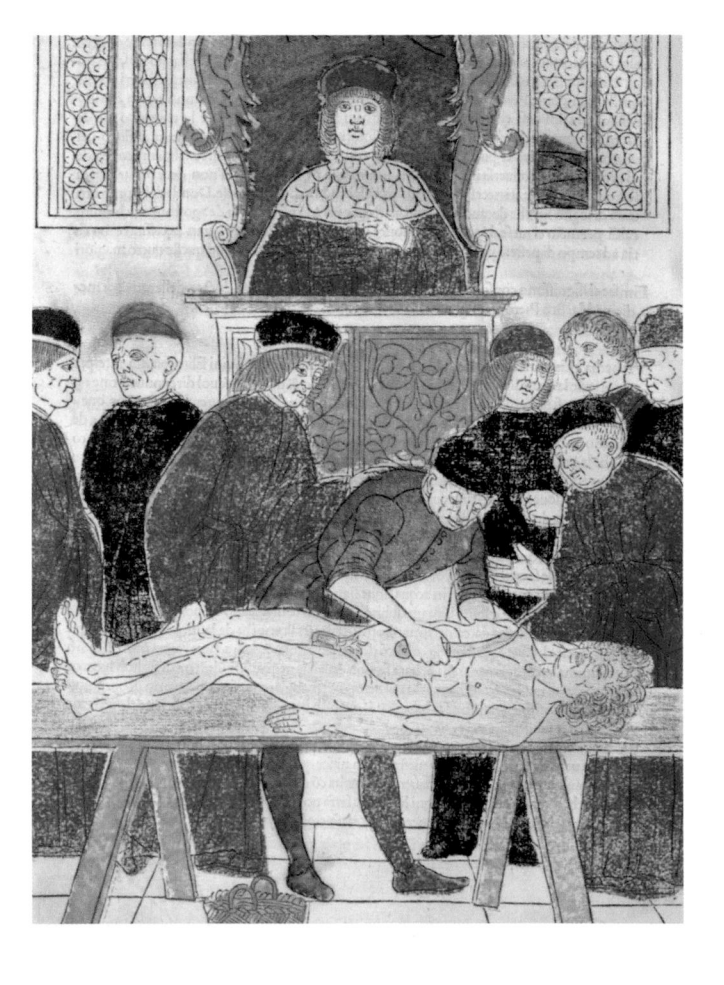

This fifteenth-century Italian picture shows the way dissections were carried out before the days of Vesalius. The Professor of Medicine supervises but does not actually undertake the dissection himself – this was done by the surgeon. Compare the role of the physician here with the picture on page 14.

Correcting Galen

Vesalius' book *The Fabric of the Human Body* provided a comprehensive description of human anatomy. He numbered or gave letters to the illustrations so that the reader could link them to the text. In most details Vesalius showed that Galen's work was accurate, but he was not afraid to identify where Galen had been wrong.

The title page of *The Fabric of the Human Body* by Vesalius. Vesalius is shown dissecting the body himself, unlike the physician in the picture on page 13.

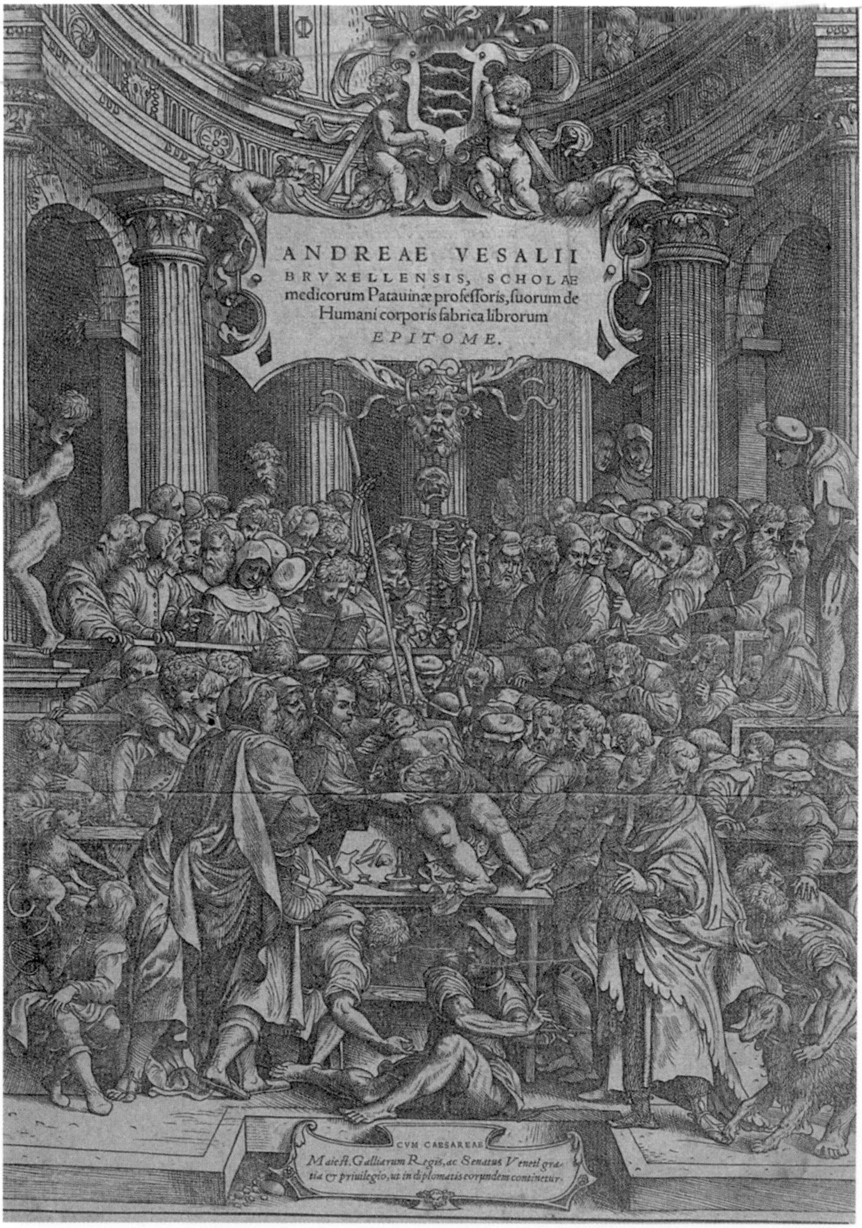

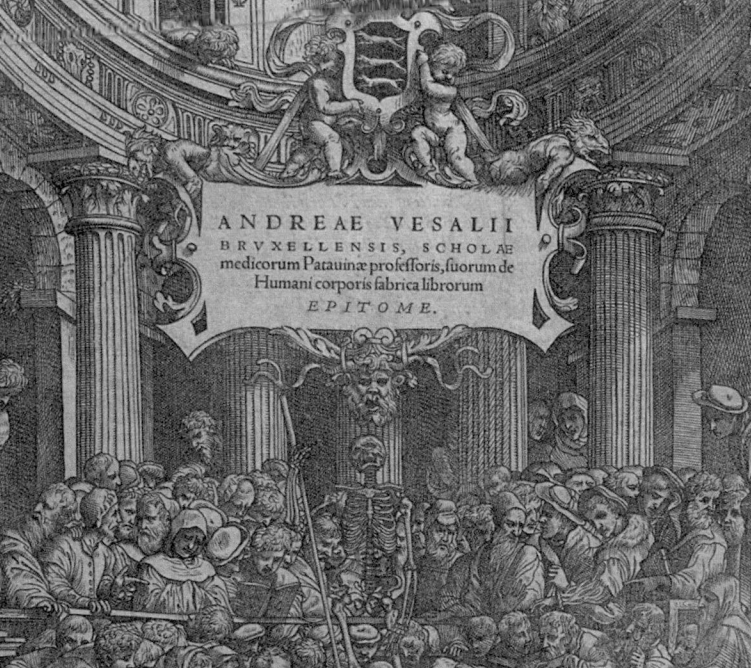

Correcting Galen was the most controversial part of Vesalius' work. Originally, Vesalius accepted Galen's descriptions of the human body and produced drawings to illustrate Galen's ideas. However, the more dissections he carried out, the more he had doubts about some details of Galen's work, because Galen's conclusions had largely been based upon his dissections of apes and pigs. By proving that Galen had been wrong about, for example, the human jaw-bone and the septum in the middle of the heart (see page 18), Vesalius encouraged other doctors to carry out their own dissections and investigations.

Art, printing and Vesalius

Vesalius' ideas spread rapidly because of developments in printing and art. At Padua in Italy he met artists who had dissected bodies and one of his own countrymen, Jan van Calcar, drew some of the illustrations for Vesalius. Vesalius also had his book printed in Basle, Switzerland by Johannes Oporinus, who was famed for his skills in book design and for the care he took over the detail in illustrations. Vesalius himself spent months in Basle checking the woodcut illustrations because, for the first time in history, they were a vital part of a medical book.

An anatomical illustration from *The Fabric of the Human Body*. Vesalius' book contained 23 full-page anatomical illustrations and another 180 smaller illustrations.

Galen can be wrong!

One of the anatomical details on which Vesalius corrected Galen was the formation of the human jaw. Vesalius wrote:

The jaw of most animals is formed of two bones joined together at the apex of the chin where the lower jaw ends in a point. In man, however, the lower jaw is formed of a single bone ... Galen and most of the skilled dissectors after the time of Hippocrates asserted that the jaw is not a single bone. However this may be, so far no human jaw has come to my attention constructed of two bones.

Paracelsus versus Galen

Despite Vesalius' correction of aspects of Galen's descriptions, sixteenth-century physicians still had great respect for the writings of Galen. However, one contemporary of Vesalius treated Galen with no respect at all. This was Paracelsus (1493–1541), the town doctor in Basle in Switzerland. He had an entirely different set of theories, declaring that Hippocrates and Galen had been wrong about most aspects of medicine.

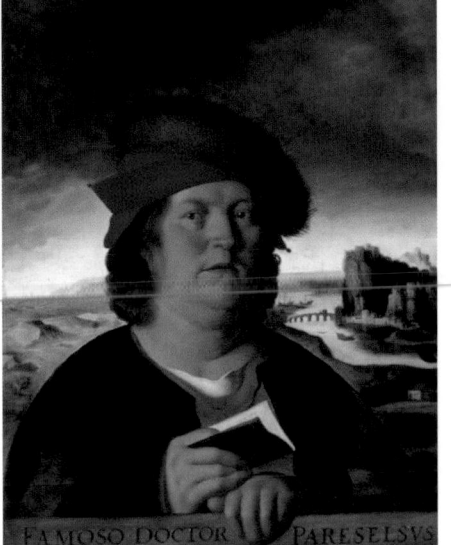

Two aspects of Paracelsus' work were revolutionary. Most dramatically, he opposed learning from books and even burned Galen's books in public to show the seriousness of his belief. He said doctors should learn through experience, at the bedsides of their patients, rather than spending their time in libraries. He also believed that God had made physicians and given them their skills, so a true physician should live and act like Jesus Christ in order to use his God-given skills effectively.

Paracelsus' religious beliefs also led him to argue for a new approach to medicine. He believed that God had created human beings and other creatures, using natural substances such as salt and other minerals, and that God had provided all the cures for illnesses in natural substances such as herbs, vegetables and minerals. Therefore he advocated that physicians should use

Paracelsus' real name was Philippus Aureolus Theophrastus Bombastus von Hohenheim, but he changed it to Paracelsus, which means 'better than Celsus'. Celsus was a renowned Roman doctor and, by choosing this name, Paracelsus was showing what he thought about the ideas of ancient medicine.

'Patients are the only books'

Two quotations from Paracelsus sum up his attitude to Galen and to other scholars (Avicenna was the European name for the great Arab medical scholar, Ibn Sina):

Galen is a liar and a fake. Avicenna is a kitchen master. They are good for nothing. You will not need them. Reading never made a doctor. Patients are the only books.

I tell you, one hair on my neck knows more than all you authors, and my shoe-buckles contain more wisdom than both Galen and Avicenna.

natural cures and he rejected the theory of the Four Humours as an explanation for illness and the treatments based on the theory.

As a result of his rejection of Galen, Paracelsus was fiercely criticized by influential university physicians. However, the religious and natural aspects of his ideas appealed to some physicians and many patients. Some physicians did use his methods, including some royal doctors such as the physician to Emperor Rudolf II of Austria. The work of Paracelsus demonstrated the divide between the old theories supported in the universities and the new ideas that appealed to patients and those physicians who were prepared to challenge the old ideas.

Local surgeons used tried and tested methods. This painting by Adriaen Brouwer (1605–1638) shows a local surgeon treating a farmer's leg. Everyday medicine was worlds apart from the theoretical arguments of university physicians about the causes of illness.

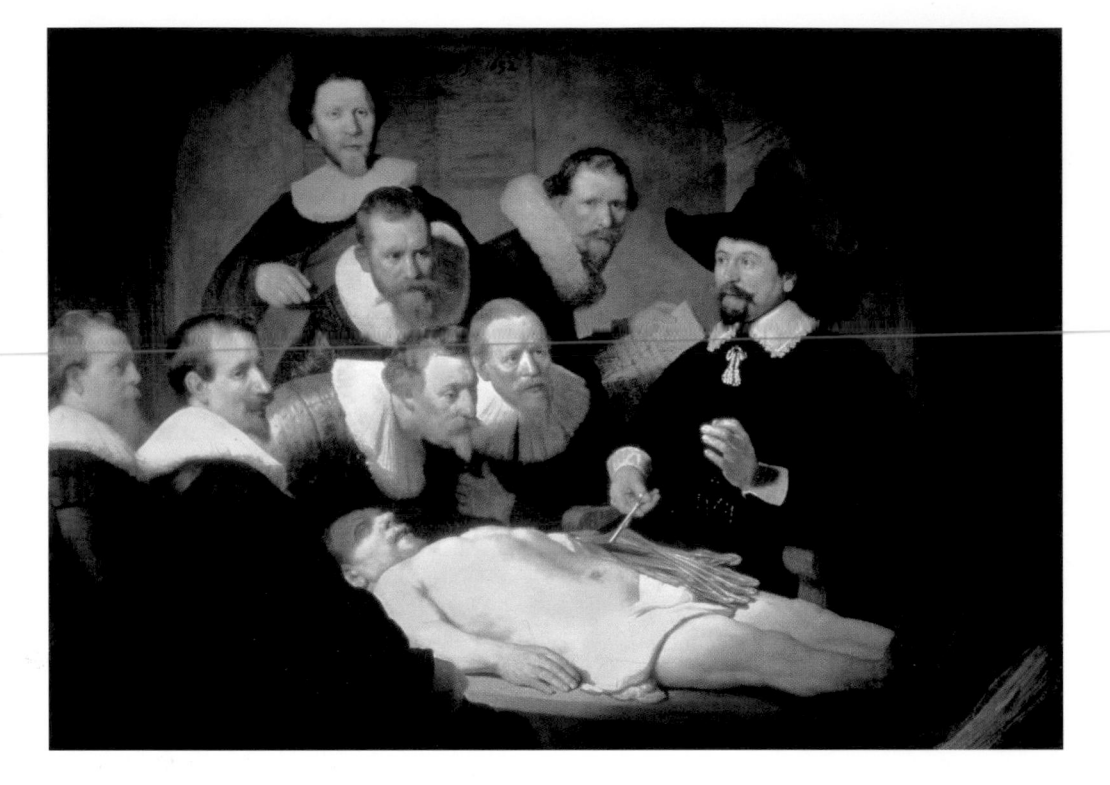

William Harvey and the circulation of the blood

One of Vesalius' key discoveries in the 1530s was that Galen had been wrong when he said that blood moves from one side of the heart to the other through holes in the septum, a membrane in the middle of the heart. Vesalius showed that there were no holes in the septum, which raised the question… "how does blood move around the body?"

During the rest of the sixteenth century, other anatomists explored this question. Now that Vesalius had built up a good general description of human anatomy, other medical scientists took over, investigating each organ in more and more detail. Realdo Columbo (c. 1515–1559) from Italy proved that blood moved from one side of the heart to the other through the lungs and Fabricius (c. 1533–1619), also from Italy, made a detailed study of the valves in veins. William Harvey, an English doctor and scientist who had been a pupil of Fabricius at the University of Padua,

By the 1600s, universities in northern Europe had followed developments in Italy and Spain and were teaching anatomy using dissection rather than simply from books. This painting is *The Anatomy Lesson of Dr Nicolaes Tulp* by the Dutch artist Rembrandt (1608–1669).

continued their work. Harvey finally proved that blood is pumped around the body by the heart, publishing his discovery in *An Anatomical Account of the Motion of the Heart and Blood in Animals* in 1628. In so doing, Harvey confirmed the work of the Arab scholar Ibn al-Nafis (1200–1288), who had theorized that blood circulated around the body, but no one had followed up his ideas.

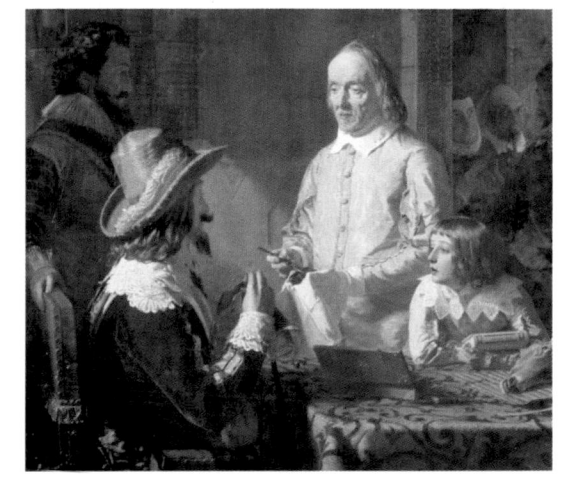

How did Harvey make his discovery?

Harvey's discovery was the result of careful dissection, observation of detail and experiment. The first stage of discovery came when Harvey noticed that the valves in the veins only allowed blood to flow *towards* the heart and that valves in the arteries only permitted blood to flow *away* from the heart. "Why did these valves only work one way?" he thought. Next, Harvey calculated the amount of blood going into the arteries each hour. Astonishingly, this amounted to three times the weight of a man. Where did all this blood come from and where was it going?

Harvey explaining the circulation of the blood to King Charles I. This painting is by Robert Hannah in 1848.

William Harvey 1578–1657

For all his brilliance, Harvey was a short-tempered man who always wore a dagger! Educated at universities in Paris and Padua, he became Chief Physician at St Bartholomew's Hospital, London in 1607, where he had to spend at least one day a week treating the poor as well as his own private patients. Later he became a royal doctor, travelling with Charles I during the Civil War but continuing his experiments and dissections whenever he got the chance. He summed up his approach to medical study with the words, "I prefer to learn and teach anatomy not from books but from dissections."

Galen must be wrong

Galen had said that excess blood was consumed by the body, but Harvey deduced that this theory must be wrong. He felt that it could not possibly explain the disappearance of so much blood. Harvey based his conclusions on dissections of human bodies and on vivisection of live animals such as frogs. He carefully noted the quantity of blood being pumped by the heart in an hour, compared it with the quantity of blood in the whole body and realized that more blood was being pumped in the hour than was actually in the whole body! This could only be explained if the blood coming from the heart was the same blood, being measured several times in the hour. Harvey concluded it was being pumped around the body by the heart. He then established that the blood firstly moves away from the heart along the arteries and then back to the heart along the veins, thanks to those one-way valves he had discovered earlier.

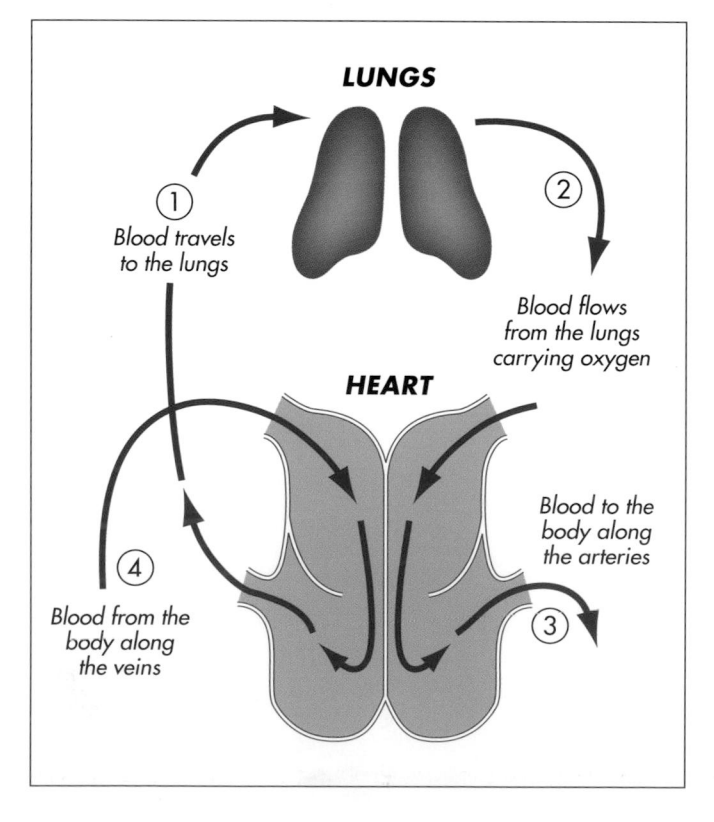

This diagram shows a simplified version of the circulation of the blood. It leaves the heart (1), passes through the lungs (2) and then flows through the body along the arteries (3) before returning to the heart along the veins (4). Then the cycle begins again.

LUNGS

① Blood travels to the lungs

② Blood flows from the lungs carrying oxygen

HEART

Blood to the body along the arteries

④ Blood from the body along the veins

③

The first microscopes

Harvey's discovery laid the groundwork for other scientists' investigations of physiology. Harvey could not, for example, explain how blood moves from the arteries to the veins. In 1660, Professor Marcello Malphigi, who was working in Bologna, Italy saw, for the first time, the capillaries, which lie close to the surface of the lungs and link the arteries to the veins. The capillaries are invisible to the naked eye, but Malphigi was using one of the earliest effective microscopes. "I could clearly see", wrote Malphigi in excitement, "that the blood flows through tortuous vessels." The great Italian scientist Galileo had developed a microscope in the 1620s, but the real breakthrough came in the 1660s when effective microscopes were produced by several scientists, including Malphigi, Antoni van Leeuwenhoek, a Dutch clothier and amateur instrument-maker, and Robert Hooke, an English scientist.

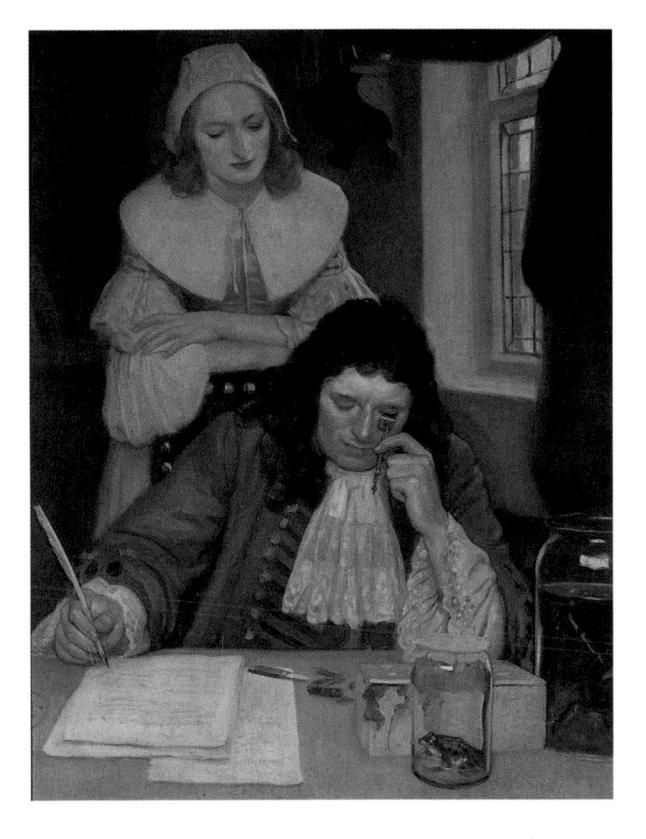

Antoni van Leeuwenhoek was the first man to use a microscope to see 'animalcules' (later known as bacteria and other organisms) in liquids, although he did not understand their significance in medicine.

Robert Hooke's *Micrographia*

In 1665 Robert Hooke published his book, *Micrographia*, which was written in English, not Latin, so that more people could read it. His book described the discoveries he made using a microscope and it provided clear illustrations, many of which were drawn by Christopher Wren, the architect who designed St Paul's Cathedral. Hooke described and pictured the structure of feathers, the nature of a butterfly's wing, the structure of the eye of a fly and numerous other details of living creatures that had never been described or illustrated before. This book almost literally opened people's eyes to the possibilities of what could be discovered by using a microscope and led to considerable further scientific enquiry.

Chapter 3

Who could you go to if you were ill?

Women in medicine

If you fell ill during this period you would probably have turned first to the women of your family. Throughout Europe, women played a major part in everyday medicine, nursing the sick and mixing herbal remedies. Wealthy ladies were often educated in how to provide medical care for local families. Lady Grace Mildmay (1552–1620), for example, was required by her governess to read William Turner's book *A New Herbal* and she continued to read widely, including books on surgery. She kept records of her patients and the treatments she used. These show she was well acquainted with the writings of Galen, the Arab scholar Ibn Sina and with Paracelsus.

A midwife delivers a baby in an illustration from a book by Jacob Rueff in 1554. Its Latin title translates as *The Conception and Birth of Humans*.

Women, midwifery and a secret

Many women throughout Europe were practising midwives. They were expected to obtain licences from the local bishop and take an oath promising not to practise witchcraft or demand high fees. There was great concern about witchcraft, particularly in the Church, and elderly single women often had to deal with accusations of being a witch.

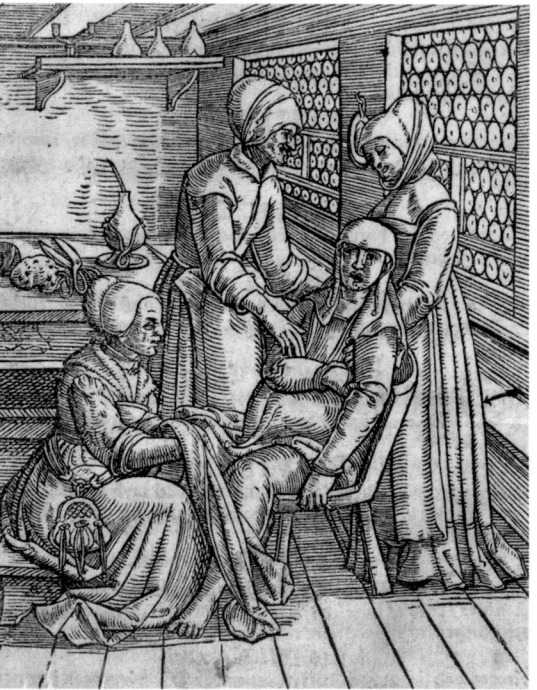

However, many women were highly respected, none more so than a German midwife, Margarita Fuss (1555–1626). Margarita was trained by her mother, who was also a midwife, and studied in Cologne and Strasbourg. She worked throughout Germany, Holland and Denmark. When she died, cathedral bells were rung in honour of 'Mother Greta', as she was known.

The use of forceps

One thing midwives did not know was that a vital piece of equipment, the obstetrical forceps, had been invented but was being kept secret by its inventors. They used the forceps to free a baby from the womb during a difficult birth without harming the baby or mother. The inventors were members of the Chamberlen family, French refugees living in England from the late 1500s. The design was passed from father to son, until the death of the last member of the family in 1728 revealed their secret. No one had seen the forceps because women were fully covered during childbirth by a sheet for the sake of decency and so no one could see exactly how the Chamberlens dealt with difficult births!

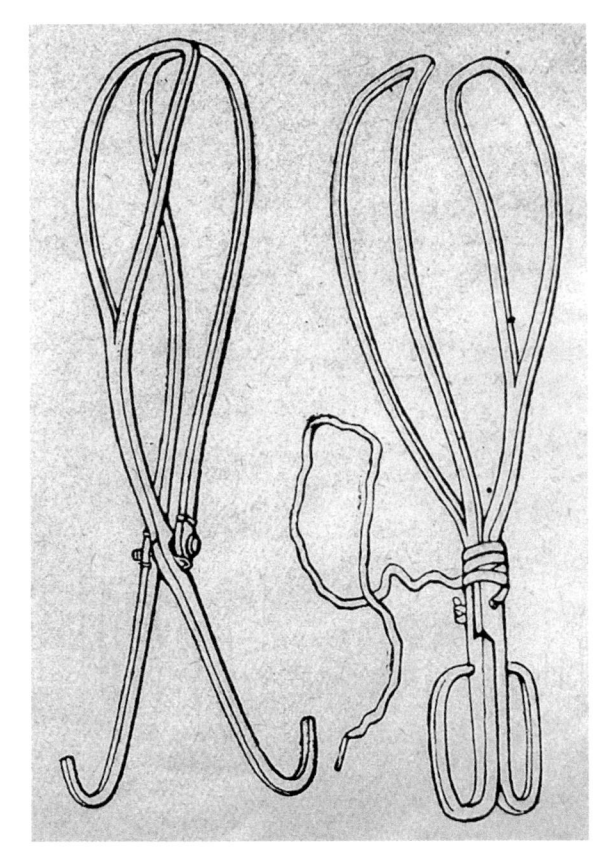

The obstetric forceps invented by the Chamberlen family, which have saved the lives of many babies and mothers. In 1818 a box containing what were probably the original forceps was found underneath the floor of a house that had belonged to the family.

The influence of one midwife

One of the most influential midwives was a Frenchwoman, Louise Bourgoise (1563–1636). Louise was married to one of the assistants of the leading French surgeon, Ambroise Paré (see page 43), and she learnt some of her medical skills from the great surgeon. She worked as a midwife to noble families and wrote a comprehensive book on obstetrics, which was published in 1609. One of her valuable suggestions was giving iron supplements to pregnant women to reduce the chances of anaemia, caused by a lack of iron in the blood. Her book was translated into four other languages. Partly as a result of her influence, midwives in Paris received formal training at the Hôtel Dieu, the great city hospital. Later, in 1679, midwives in Amsterdam followed the French example by attending lectures on anatomy and obstetrics.

Physicians and their training

If home remedies did not immediately cure an illness, then wealthy families could call in a university-trained physician to visit them in their home. University training took at least six years and often longer if a student decided to study at a famous medical school, such as those at Bologna or Padua in Italy or Montpellier in France. Students did spend some time observing the work of an experienced physician, but most of their studies involved reading the writings of Greek and Roman doctors, particularly Hippocrates and Galen, just as it had done in the Middle Ages.

When Harvey discovered the circulation of the blood, his findings were initially greeted with hostility by many university physicians because he was contradicting Galen. Some simply ignored Harvey's theory. Others argued that he must be wrong. His discovery was only gradually accepted. It was not until 1673, nearly 50 years after Harvey published his evidence, that the teachers at the University of Paris taught Harvey's ideas rather than Galen's.

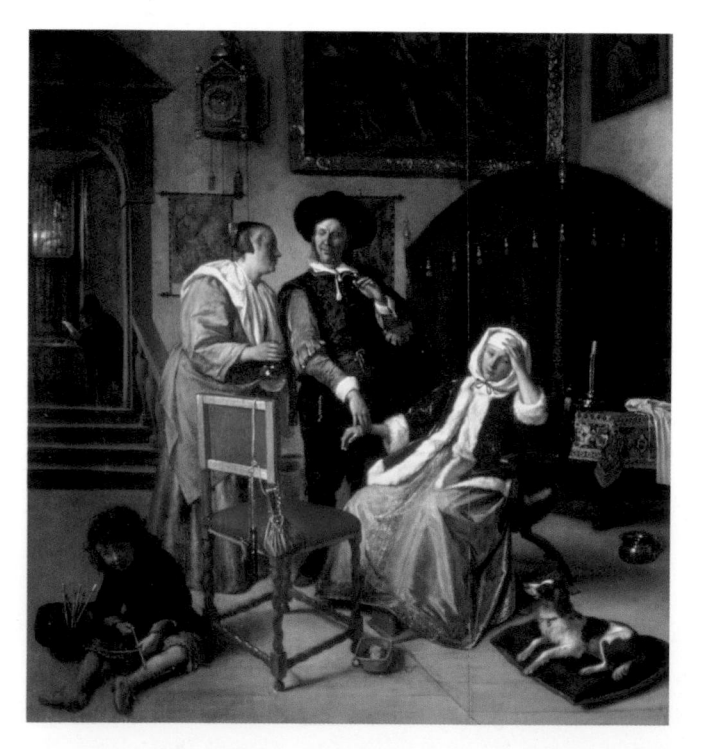

A painting entitled *The Doctor's Visit* by Jan Steen, dating from *c.* 1663. The physician is visiting his wealthy patient at home. After all their years of training, physicians expected to live comfortably off the fees paid by their wealthy patients. Becoming a royal doctor was the height of their ambition.

Duties to their patients

One of the main duties of physicians to their patients was to advise them on how to stay healthy through eating a good diet and taking exercise, just as their ancient and medieval predecessors had done. If a patient became ill, then physicians diagnosed the precise malady by inspecting the patient's urine and consulting astrological charts. Their treatments were still based on Hippocrates' theory that illness was caused by an imbalance in the body's humours. They therefore recommended treatments that would restore a healthy balance, such as bleeding and purging, which emptied the bowels. Despite the medical discoveries of Vesalius and others, the day-to-day work of a physician had changed little since the Middle Ages.

Uroscopy, examining the appearance of urine, was one of the most common means of diagnosing illness in the sixteenth and seventeenth centuries. This scene would have been familiar to anyone visiting a physician.

Doctor or wisewoman?

By the 1680s it was very fashionable to see a university-educated doctor, but not everyone agreed that doctors' qualifications were useful. John Aubrey, an English writer who lived up to the late 1600s, recorded the views of Thomas Hobbes on such fashionable doctors:

Hobbes is regarded as one of the greatest philosophers to have lived. Mr Hobbes used to say that he had rather have the advice or take medicine from an experienced old woman, who had been at many sick people's bedsides, than from the learnedst but unexperienced physician.

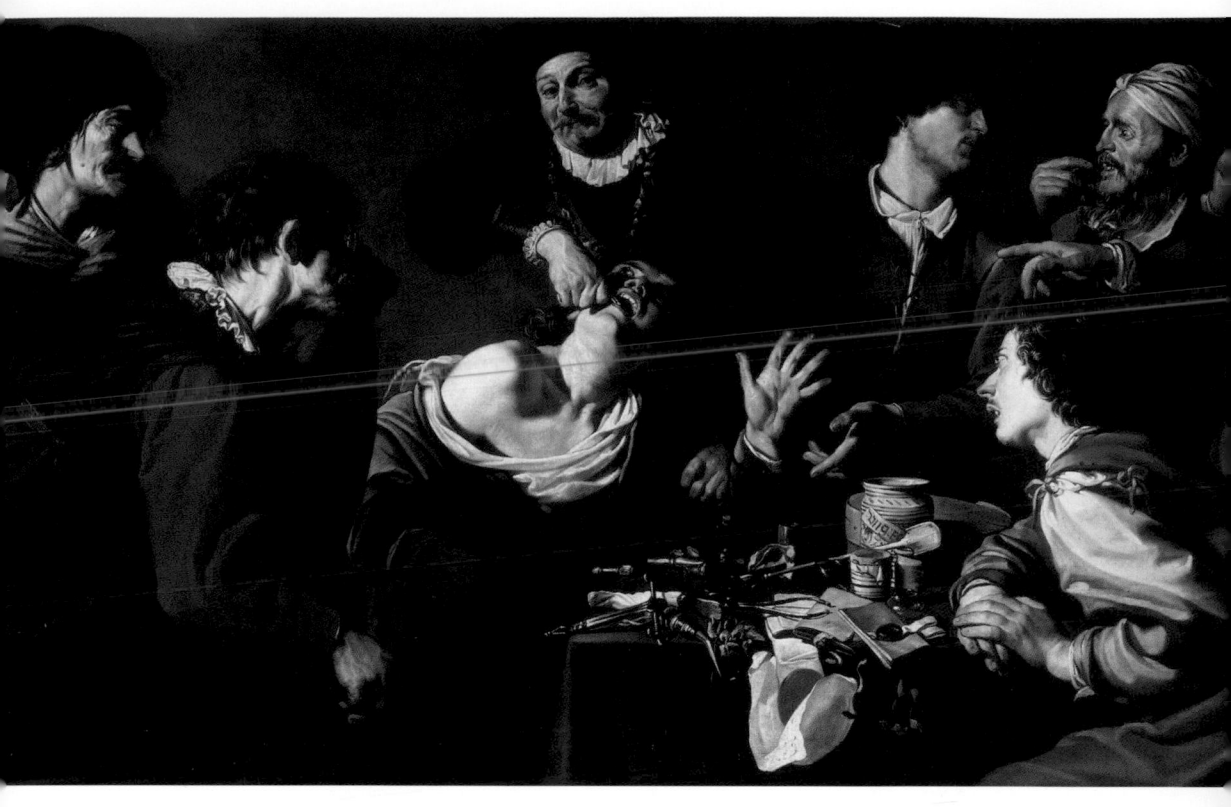

The fight for medical supremacy

If you were ill and could not afford to pay to see a physician then you could visit a barber-surgeon (see page 40) or an apothecary. In the eyes of the physicians, both these kinds of healers were inferior because they had not been university-trained and knew little of the writings of Galen and the other ancient authors. The physicians endeavoured to take control of the surgeons and apothecaries. They wanted to stipulate who had the right to provide medical help and so limit the impact of the surgeons and apothecaries on their own practice. They also tried to exclude women from working as healers, even as midwives.

However, despite their best efforts, the physicians failed to dominate medicine because ordinary people were extremely sceptical of their theories and treatments and frequently preferred the more familiar remedies and potions available from surgeons and apothecaries. Even the greatest physicians were not

A toothpuller at work *c.* 1620, an example of a medical treatment that nearly everyone needed but everyone tried to avoid in the days before anaesthetics.

respected by their social inferiors. William Harvey lamented that after he published his book on the circulation of the blood, fewer patients came to see him and many thought he was mad.

Physicians could not even agree amongst themselves. While university professors insisted on the importance of reading and theory, Thomas Sydenham, one of the most respected physicians in late seventeenth-century London, advocated: "Young man, you must go to the bedside. It is there alone that you can learn about disease".

Sydenham stressed that doctors needed to take a full history of the patient's health and symptoms at the bedside, observing and recording the illness with great care. He wrote: "I have been very careful to write nothing but what was the product of faithful observation and neither suffered myself to be deceived by idle speculations nor have deceived others by obtruding anything upon them but downright matters of fact."

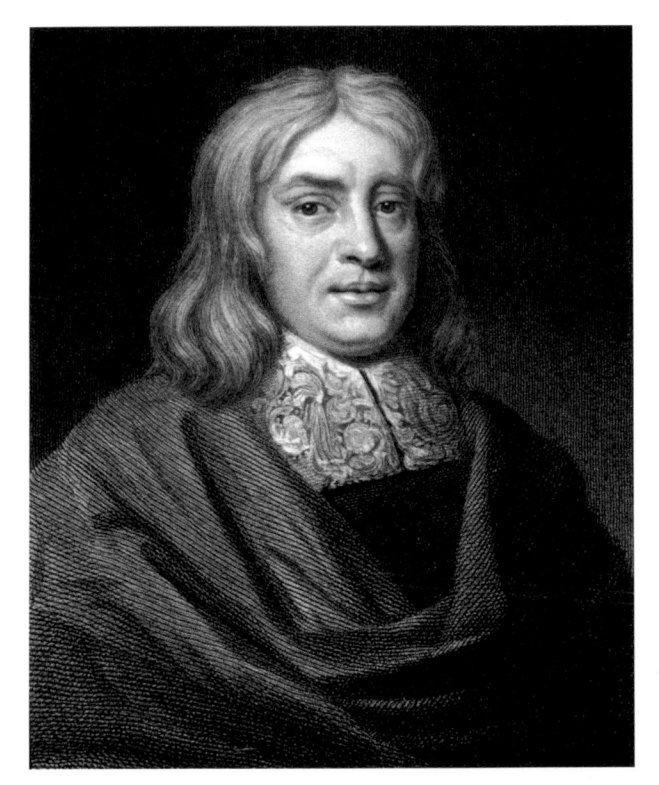

Thomas Sydenham (1624–1689). Sydenham's practical approach to medicine may have developed because he spent several years fighting in the English Civil War and so spent less time at university.

The 'English Hippocrates'

Thomas Sydenham became known as the 'English Hippocrates' because the legendary Greek doctor had placed great importance on careful observation of patients, as did Sydenham. Sydenham's observations contributed to medical knowledge because he made detailed descriptions of many illnesses, including the first description of scarlet fever. He believed that each disease was distinctly different and that it was important to identify the exact disease so that the correct remedy could be chosen to cure it. He also believed in allowing the body to fight the illness by itself. Patients who were used to physicians ordering bleeding or purging must have been delighted when Sydenham prescribed roast chicken and a bottle of wine to restore their strength!

Apothecaries

Apothecaries were found in towns all over Europe, selling herbal remedies and other drugs at their shops. Apothecaries made up prescriptions for physicians or sold their own medicines directly to the public. They also performed low-level medical tasks, such as 'drawing' (pulling out) teeth. Although physicians regarded apothecaries as inferior, they won great respect during the Great Plague of London because most stayed in London when the physicians fled to the countryside! In country areas they were often the most qualified medical men, especially if they belonged to an organization that regulated their work. For example, the Society of Apothecaries, founded in 1617, made sure that its London members kept to its regulations and maintained good standards.

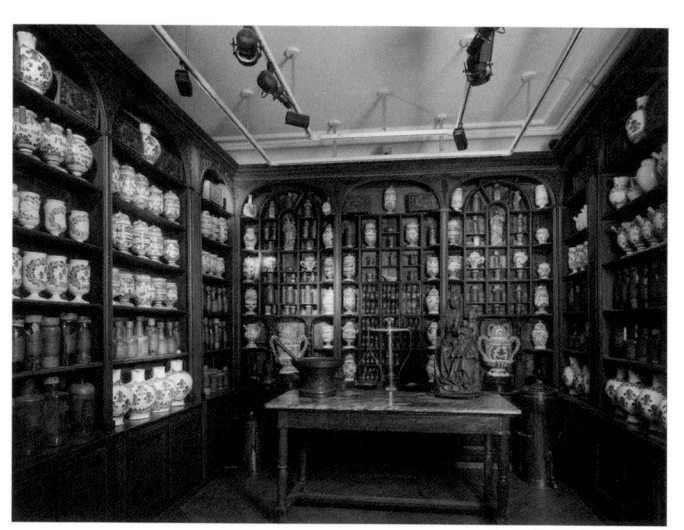

A particularly grand apothecary's shop in seventeenth-century Paris. There was an extremely wide range of herbs and other items on sale, from honey (which had been used since the era of the Ancient Egyptians to combat infections) to exotics such as powdered rhinoceros horn.

Quacks

Quacks were healers who had no professional training, travelling sellers of medicines 'guaranteed' to make you feel better! Some quacks did help the sick because they were selling herbal remedies that had been developed through trial and error over many decades. Others were simply out to make money, arriving in town with a fanfare of drum and trumpet, accompanied by a capering clown and chattering monkey to draw in the

Trash medicines

A pamphlet written around 1670 warned people about the dangers of listening to quacks and being taken in by long words:

When people tell him their griefs and their ills, though he knows not what ails them any more than if they were a horse, he tells them it is a scorbutic humour caused by a defluxion from the os-scarum, afflicting the diaphiaragma and circoary-thenordal muscles. The poor souls are abundantly satisfied with this and are amazed that he's hit on their problem so exactly. He has an excellent talent for persuading well people that they are sick and giving them his trash medicines soon makes this come true.

A quack at work selling medicines in the town square in Mantua, Italy c. 1520.

crowds. Some even pretended to be from faraway places, such as Turkey, to add a sense of mystery and excitement.

Some earned quite a bit of money. One English quack, Joanna Stephens who lived during the 1700s, claimed to have developed a remedy that would dissolve bladder stones without the patient needing a painful operation (see pages 38–39). Parliament paid £5000 to buy the recipe from her! Cornelius Tilburg, a Dutch quack of the late 1600s, claimed his secret potion was an antidote to poisons and could cure blindness, deafness and many other ailments. Both rich and poor bought medicines from the quacks, revealing perhaps what little confidence they had in the treatments on offer from the physicians.

Chapter 4

How did they treat the sick?

Home remedies

Throughout Europe, home remedies were handed down through the generations from mother to daughter. Girls learned how to mix up remedies, using ingredients such as honey which, experience showed, prevented infection. Modern experiments have shown such remedies to be effective, even if people did not know the scientific basis of the treatments at the time.

We have further evidence of home remedies from the sixteenth century onwards. More people had learned to read and write and so were able to write down their remedies. Mary Doggett, the wife of a London actor, described remedies for ailments such as colic, jaundice and even plague. For scurvy, she used a mixture, taken two or three times a day, of horseradish roots, white wine, water and a quart (just over a litre) of orange juice or twelve thinly cut oranges. Scurvy, a disease that leads to internal bleeding and death, results from not eating enough fruit and vegetables – people do not take in enough vitamin C. Mary did not know that this was the reason, simply that this mixture worked wonders!

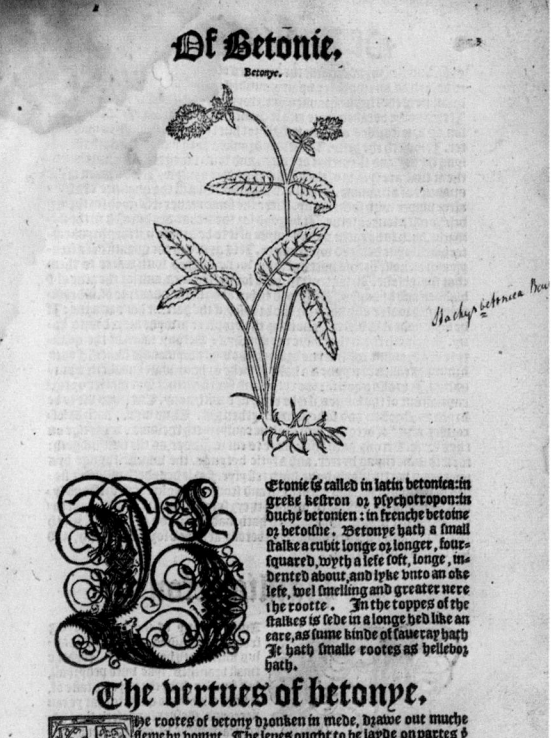

A page from William Turner's *New Herbal*, published in 1551. This page describes the uses of the plant called betony, whose roots could be mixed with honey to make a drink that was used to bring up phlegm.

Herbs, mercury and human skull

More complex home remedies were available from women who specialized in medical treatments, such as Lady Grace Mildmay (see page 22). She developed a favourite remedy, her 'precious balm', which took five weeks to make! It included, amongst other things, 24 types of root, 68 herbs, 14 different seeds, 12 flowers, 10 spices, 20 kinds of gum, two pints (one litre) of vinegar, two gallons (9 litres) of olive oil, and six pounds (2.7 kilograms) of sugar. She used mostly herbs in her remedies, but she also used metals and minerals recommended by Paracelsus, such as amber, gold and mercury, and occasional exotic ingredients such as elk hooves, crab's claws and powder of human skull. Lady Mildmay treated skin diseases, ulcers, fevers and many other ailments among local people, who would not have revisited her if her remedies had not frequently been helpful.

One of the most popular books containing advice on herbal remedies was Nicholas Culpepper's *English Physician and Complete Herbal*, which recommended simple home-grown herbal remedies.

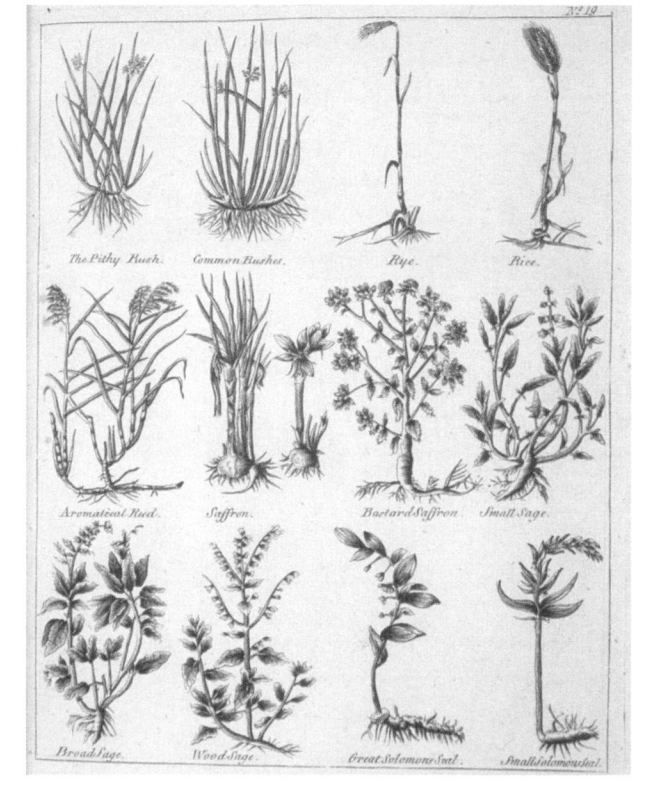

A cure for anaemia

Although Mary Doggett did not write down which problem she treated with this remedy, it would have been effective in helping people suffering from anaemia, a condition caused by a lack of iron in the blood; it particularly affects pregnant women.

To make steel wine. Take filings of steel, which you can find at the needle-makers, wash it in water to cleanse it from dust, then wet it with vinegar upon a stone for 3 or 4 days. Let it dry until it is red with rust, the more rusty and old the better, then pound it and search it very fine [to pick out remaining dirt]. Put two pounds of it in any wine. Shake it everyday for a week to mix.

New ingredients from abroad

European travels to America and Asia, beginning in the late fifteenth century, led to hopes of new, effective medicines being brought to Europe. This was based on the belief that a merciful God had given people in every country remedies to cure the diseases that were native to that country. Explorers also intended to sell the new medicines at a considerable profit.

Among the new plants to arrive in Europe was rhubarb, which was introduced from Asia in the early seventeenth century. It was widely and successfully used to purge the bowels. Another was the plant *ipecacuanha*, brought from Brazil in the late 1600s, which was used to make people vomit and was prescribed for dysentery. It is still recognized today as an effective cure for dysentery and is also still regularly used as an expectorant to clear the chest of phlegm.

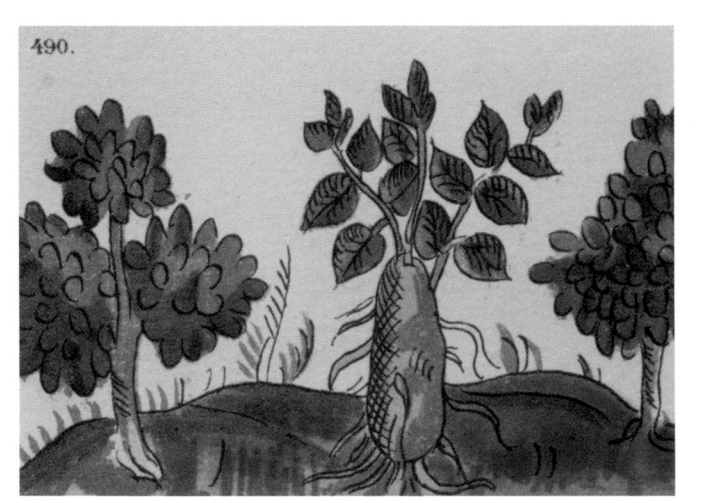

The bark of the *cinchona* tree, illustrated here in the *Florentine Codex*. This account of Aztec society was compiled *c.* 1570 by a Spanish Priest, Bernardino de Sahagun, who spent many years in Mexico. The *cinchona* tree was imported from South America because of its effectiveness in treating fevers. In Europe it became known as 'quinine' and it has helped many who suffered from malaria. It is still used today in a different form.

These and other medicines were expensive to buy in Europe, but nonetheless were very popular, partly because they were so new and exotic. Nicolas Monardes, a Spanish physician, was among the writers to popularize medicines from the Americas in books published between 1565 and 1574. His work was so well loved that it was translated from Spanish into French, German, Latin and English. The English version was entitled *Joyful News out of the New Found World*.

However, not all physicians believed that these imported medicines were useful to Europeans. Many followers of Paracelsus (page 16) turned the argument about God providing medicines against the promoters of the new medicines. The opponents of the use of foreign medicines said that God had given each region remedies for the diseases of that region. Therefore medicines from other regions would not work against local diseases. In reply, the physicians who were followers of Galen, said that diseases were universal – the same throughout the world – and cures could be found in all countries. Without detailed scientific analysis to help them, these theoretical arguments continued without a conclusion.

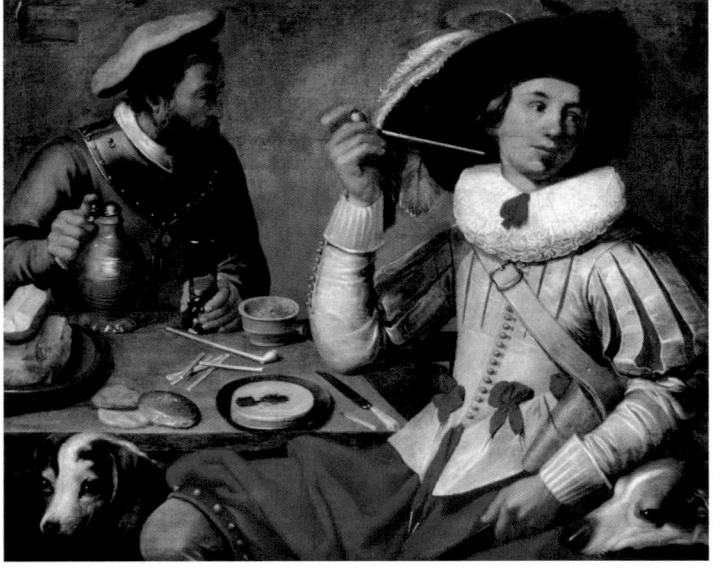

Tobacco was greeted as a cure-all when it arrived from America (see panel). People were so convinced that tobacco could protect them from the plague that schoolboys at Eton College in England were flogged during the Great Plague of 1665 if they did not smoke often enough! This painting *Two Soldiers* is by the Dutch artist Jacob Gerritzs (1594–1652).

The uses of tobacco and opium

People regarded tobacco and opium as valuable medicines long before it was discovered how much harm they did to their users. Tobacco, imported from America from the early 1600s, was recommended for toothache, poisoned wounds, joint pains, bad breath, ulcers, chilblains, tiredness and many other ailments. Opium was imported from Turkey and was used as an anaesthetic and to treat many ailments including dysentery and breathing problems. Thomas Sydenham (see page 27) proclaimed: "Among the remedies which it has pleased the Almighty God to give to man to relieve his sufferings, none is so universal and so efficacious as opium".

The fight against smallpox

Another cure to come from abroad helped in the fight against smallpox. Smallpox was a common but rarely fatal disease in sixteenth-century Europe. However, during the seventeenth century, the nature of smallpox changed, possibly because a new type of the disease arrived in Europe from Asia. From then on, frequent epidemics killed hundreds and sometimes thousands. Physicians could not agree on how to treat it and none of their methods was successful.

The first answer to smallpox arrived from Asia. Lady Mary Wortley Montagu (1689–1762) was the wife of a British diplomat in Turkey. She had watched as Turkish women held 'smallpox parties' – they brought their children to an old woman who "comes with a nutshell full of the matter of the best sort of smallpox and asks what veins you please to have open'd. She immediately rips open … and puts into the vein as much [smallpox] matter as can lie upon the head of her needle."

Back in England, Lady Mary recommended this treatment to friends who were doctors. The

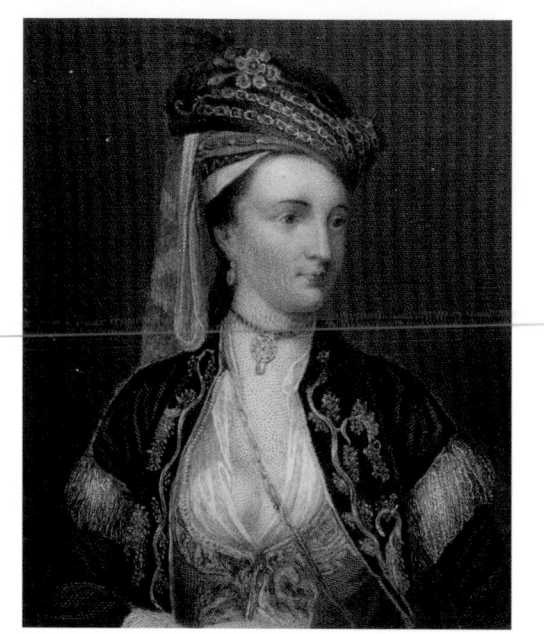

Lady Mary Wortley Montagu was so convinced of the value of inoculation that she took the risk of having her own daughter inoculated with a mild dose of smallpox in 1721.

Inoculation against smallpox

These extracts are from the diary of James Woodforde, an English vicar, 2 and 22 November, 1776:

This morning about 11 o'clock Dr Thorne came to my house and inoculated my servants Ben Legate and little Jack Wharton against smallpox … Pray god my people and all others may do well, several houses have got the smallpox at present. O Lord send thy blessing of health on all of them.

John Bowles's wife was inoculated by one Drake, formerly a sergeant in the Militia. He makes a deep incision in both arms and puts a plaister over, he gives no camomile but they take salts every morning.

'inoculation' gave children a mild dose of smallpox; most of them were healthy enough to fight off this small dosage and they never caught smallpox again. Experimental inoculations were tried on condemned criminals and gradually the idea spread. Robert Sutton and his sons, who were surgeons, claimed to have inoculated 400,000 people in 30 years, creating a successful money-making business. They charged people for the inoculation and sold their method to other doctors, but only to those living a long distance from their own Essex home so nobody could set up as rivals.

Inoculation, however, did have risks. Some people died from the small dose of smallpox given in the inoculation and sometimes the inoculation also spread the disease. So it was not universally used and the search for a safer method of prevention continued.

The Mineral Springs, **painted by Allart van Everdingen (1621–1675). Spa towns such as Bath were becoming increasingly popular by the 1700s. Wealthy people visited them to drink or bathe in the waters that were believed to improve health.**

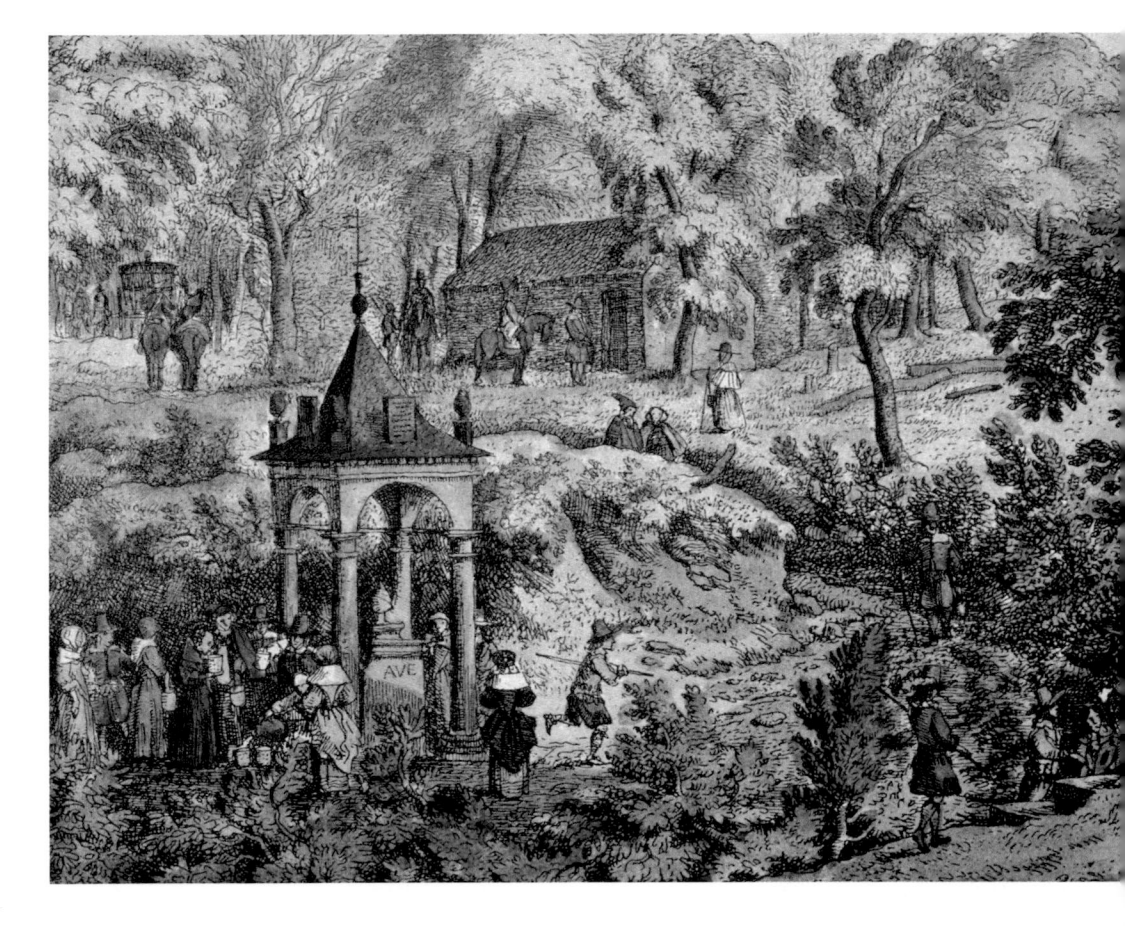

The development of hospitals

Medieval hospitals had been run by the church and were primarily rest homes for the elderly, infirm poor. They were given food and were made warm and the focus was on prayer to safeguard their souls, not medical treatment to save their bodies. Anyone with an infectious disease was not permitted to enter a hospital. This approach began to change at the end of the fifteenth century. Hospitals in Italy were the first to provide free medical treatment alongside the medieval provision of food, warmth and prayer. During the sixteenth century, hospitals in the rest of Europe began to follow this example.

Hospital records from Florence in Italy provide a clear picture of the changes taking place. By 1500, Florence had four hospitals, of which the largest, Santa Maria Nuovo, cared for over 200 people. There were male and female wards, patients received free food,

A surgeon binding up a woman's arm after she has been bled, another of the most common treatments carried out in the home and in hospitals. This painting is by Jacob Toorenvliet, 1666.

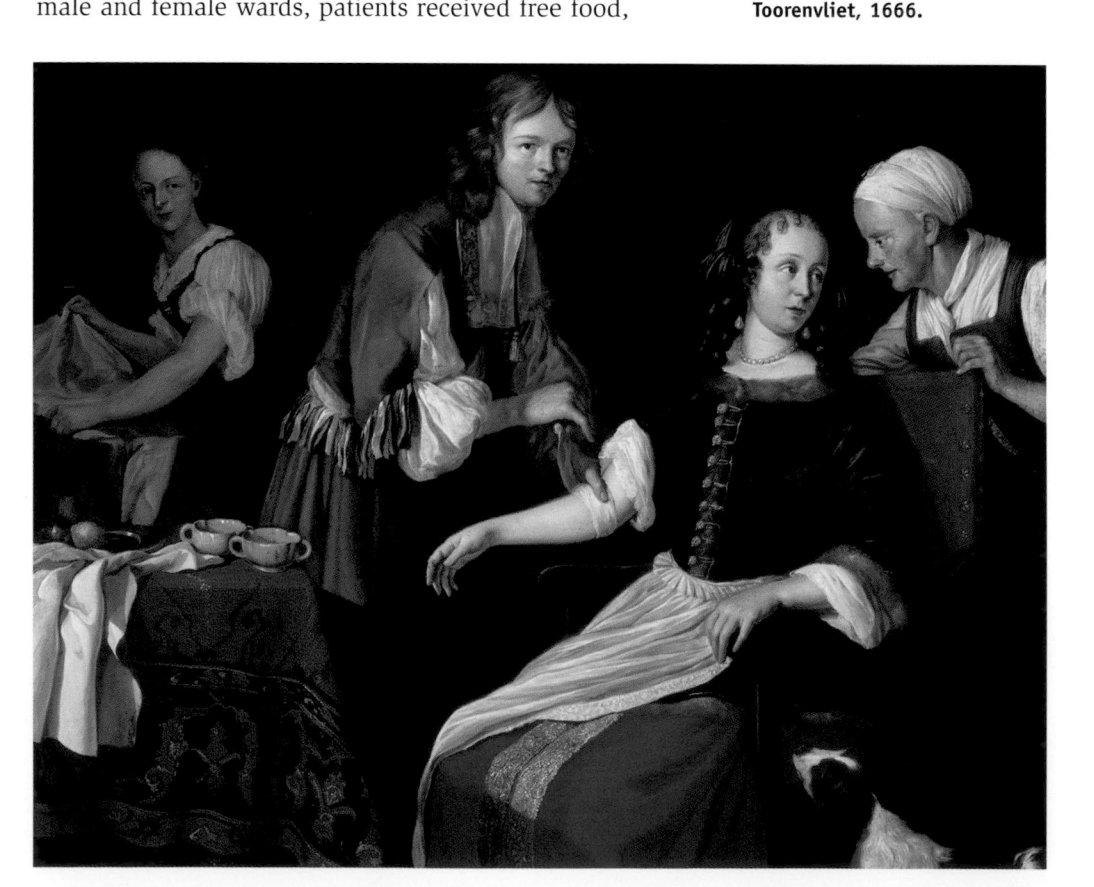

drink and medical treatment and the beds were comfortable with mattresses, pillows and linen sheets. The hospital employed ten doctors, three of whom lived at the hospital while the others visited at specific times each week. There were also surgeons and apothecaries to purchase and make drugs. The hospital was seen by doctors as a good place to learn and to develop their careers.

The hospital records show that the patients were mostly poor and they needed treatments for health problems. The male patients, in particular, had short-term, curable ailments, such as fractures, wounds, skin complaints and fevers. They stayed in the hospital for a few days or weeks. Women patients, who had a separate ward, were more likely to suffer longer-term health problems and the typical female patient seems to have been older and widowed.

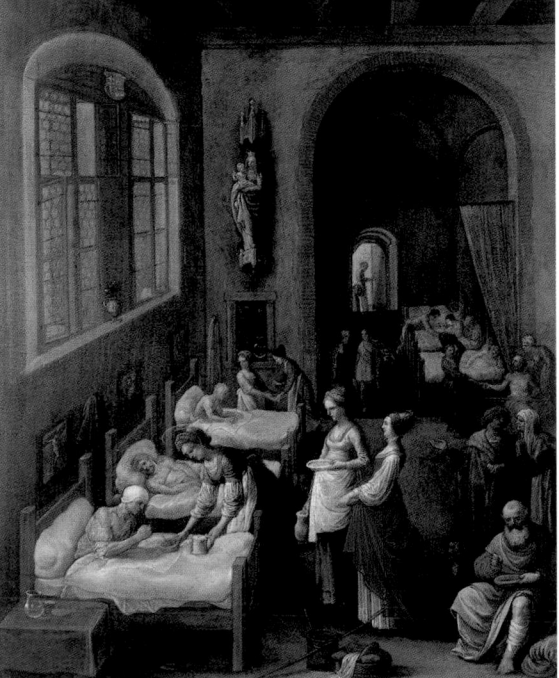

The Infirmary of the Sisters of Charity in Paris, painted in the mid-seventeenth century by Abraham Bosse (1602–1676).

Hospital rules

The following are extracts from the rules for nursing the sick at Milan's Maggiore Hospital, 1616:

As part of their duties, male nurses are to:
Provide the poor with food, distributing plums, oranges and soup at set times.
Put newcomers to bed with clean sheets.
Take note of symptoms and fevers and point these out to the physicians.
Ensure the rooms are swept twice each week.
Collect 4 clean aprons and towels each Thursday and Sunday.
Give water to the patients so they wash their hands before meals (warm water in winter).
Freshen the mouths of the patients, clean their tongues and issue chamber pots.

Chapter 5

How effective was Renaissance surgery?

The risks of surgery

On 26 March 1658, Samuel Pepys lay on a table, praying quietly, while long strips of linen were wound round his arms, legs and neck. He was being tied down in readiness for surgery. Pepys hoped the operation could cure him but knew that there was an equal chance that it would kill him.

As long as the 25-year-old Pepys could remember, he had suffered occasional excruciating pain in his bladder. Thomas Hollier, a highly experienced surgeon at St Thomas's Hospital, London, said that the pain was caused by a stone in his bladder. Recently, the pain had become more frequent and so sharp that Pepys could not prevent himself crying out when it developed. He decided to risk the operation.

The operation took place in Pepys's cousin's house, not in a hospital. He was given a herbal drink to take the edge off the pain while Dr Hollier lubricated his instruments in warm milk and oil. The surgeon then

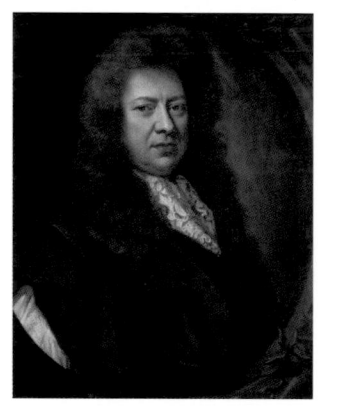

This portrait of Samuel Pepys, the famous diarist, was painted when Samuel was about 50.

Samuel Pepys 1633–1703

Pepys is famous for the fascinating diary he kept between 1660 and 1669. He described the Great Plague of 1665 and the Great Fire of London of 1666 and the diary also provides a vivid picture of the lives of ordinary Londoners. Pepys was a very able administrator, playing a vital role in building up and organizing the Royal Navy. His diary contains medical information too. For example, at the end of 1664 Pepys noted his good health but was unsure why he was so healthy, writing that he "was at a loss to know whether it [is because of] my hare's foot, or taking every morning of a pill of turpentine, or my having left off the wearing of a gown."

picked up his scalpel and made a three-inch (7.6 cm) cut, deep enough to reach the bladder and pull out the stone with forceps. He worked fast, both to save his patient pain and to reduce the chances of damaging other organs if Pepys moved at the wrong moment.

The operation over, the wound was not stitched but allowed to heal naturally. After a week, Pepys was allowed out of bed and five weeks later he felt fully recovered. He had survived the extremely risky experience of surgery! For the rest of his life Pepys celebrated the anniversary of his operation as if it was his birthday. He kept the stone in a case. It weighed two ounces (50 grams) and was almost as large as a tennis ball. That year, Hollier performed 30 successful operations, but the next year his first four patients died. Pepys was lucky because Hollier used new instruments that had not yet become infected during operations.

In this painting a surgeon operates on a man's scalp. The greatest danger of operations was that the patient developed an infection, caught from the surgeon's instruments, hands or clothes.

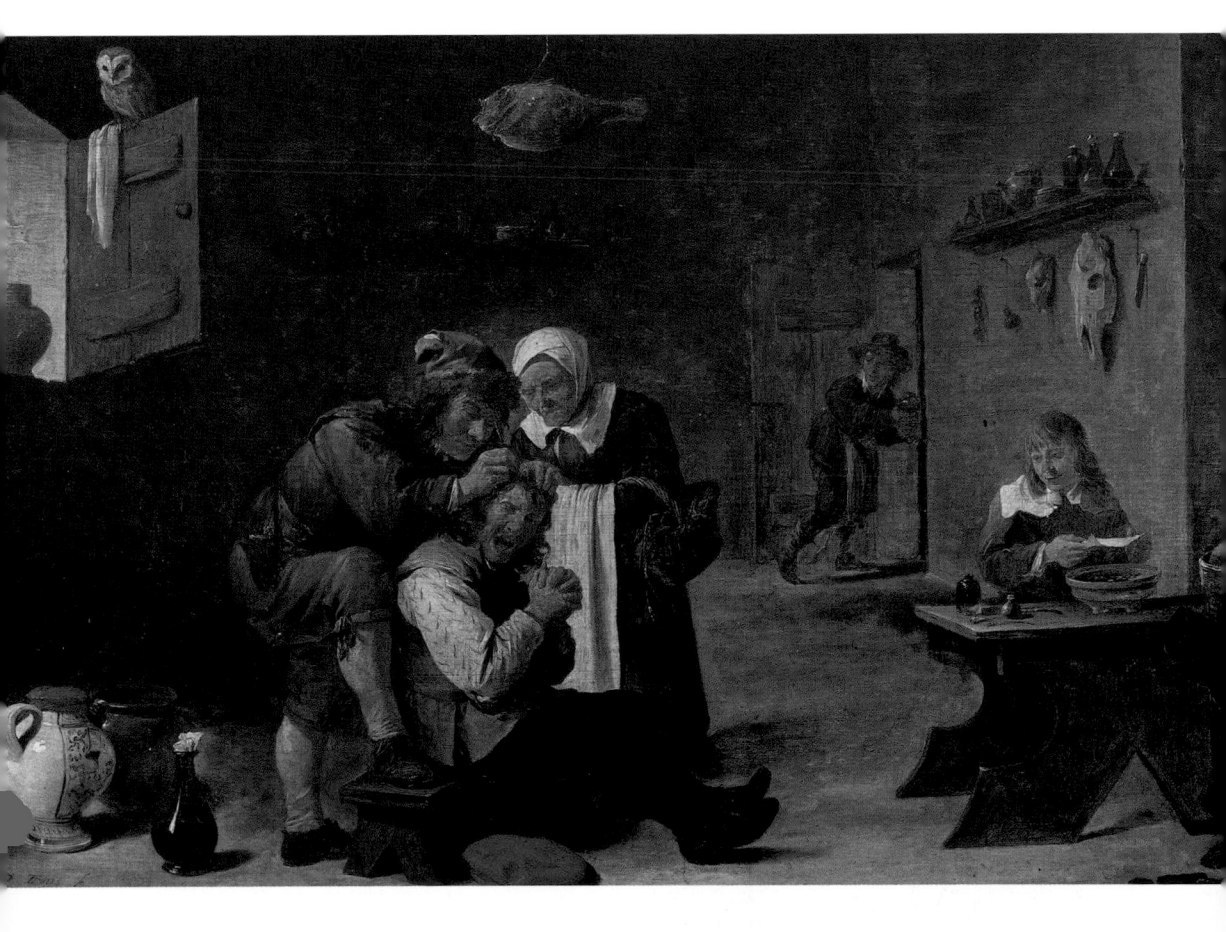

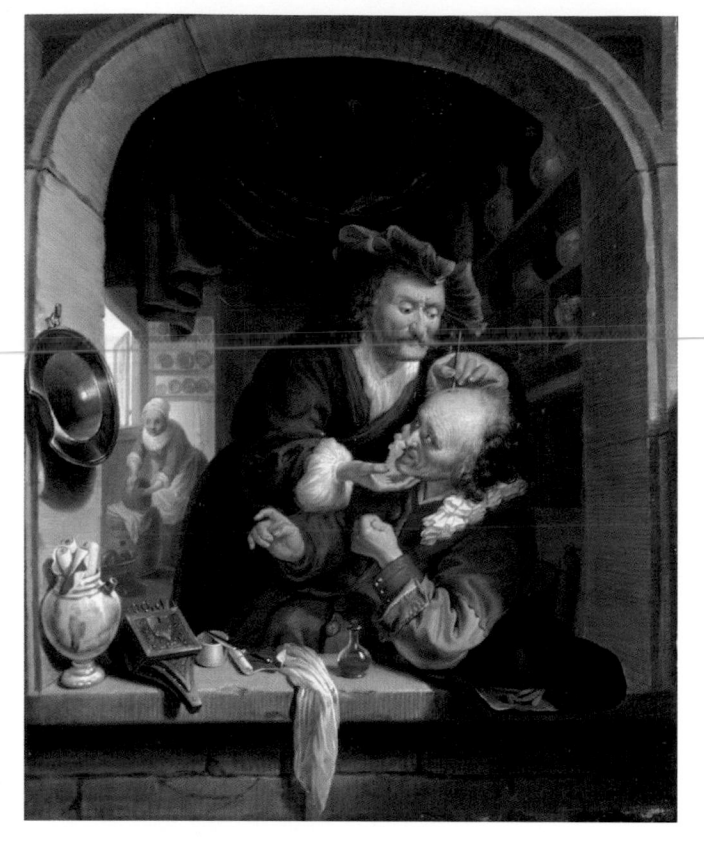

The most common providers of surgery were the barber-surgeons, so called because they mixed hair-cutting and shaving with bleeding, tooth-pulling and other basic surgical tasks. Their skills varied considerably, but the better ones joined Guilds and served apprenticeships. This barber-surgeon was painted by Issac Koedyck (1616–1668).

A surgeon's case-book

Surgery, as Samuel Pepys knew only too well, was a very risky experience. One handbook for surgeons admitted that during operations "life and death do so wrestle together that no man can tell which will have the victory". However, this does not mean that surgeons were incompetent and uncaring. It was simply that surgical techniques had not developed sufficiently to enable surgeons to help all their patients.

Intelligent surgeons operated on patients whom they knew they could help. Experience enabled them to deal successfully with broken and dislocated limbs, surface tumours and swellings and cuts such as knife wounds. The notebooks of Joseph Binns, a London surgeon, record the cases of 403 patients between 1633 and 1663, of whom 265 were cured and another 62 improved in health. This amounted to a success rate of 81 per cent. The most complex internal surgery was lithotomy – the operation suffered by Pepys to remove a bladder stone – but amputations and trepanning (a procedure whereby someone cuts into the skull to relieve pressure on the brain) were also carried out as a last resort, to save life.

Surgical training

Despite their practical skills, surgeons ranked well below university-trained physicians in status. They learned from practice and experience, training as apprentices to experienced surgeons. They did use books, but they were handbooks written by surgeons, rather than the writings of Greek and Roman doctors. They were not expected to have detailed anatomical knowledge or understand the theories of Galen, although many would have done so. Records provide evidence of women working as surgeons, although sometimes this angered male surgeons who feared losing their patients to competitors. In York in 1572, Isabel Warwick was permitted to work as a surgeon because "she has the skill in the science of surgery and has done good therein", despite the objections of the city's male surgeons.

This illustration from The *Anatomical Vademecum* (handbook) is by the Swiss physician and surgeon, Johann von Muralt, and was published in 1677.

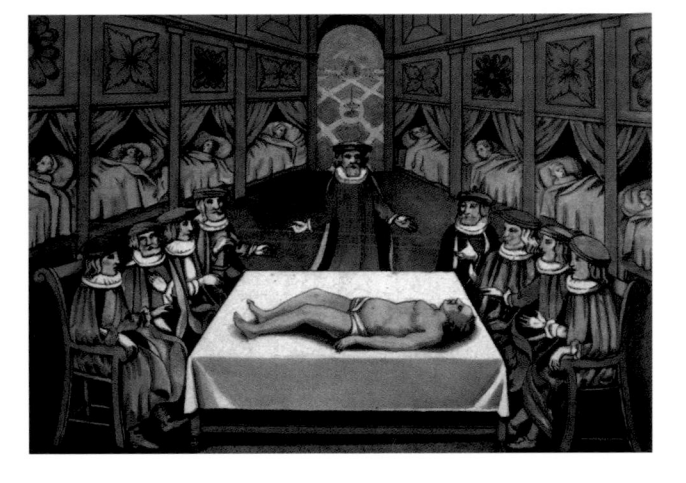

The best instructors in surgery

Richard Wiseman, surgeon to both Charles I and Charles II, was the author of two books on surgery. In the introductions he wrote:

In preparing this book I have read all the eminent surgical authors yet I have followed my own judgement and experience more than any other man's authority. Men who have spent their time working as surgeons are the best instructors. I spent my time in armies, not in universities nor books. We do not all spend our time talking in coffee houses.

Battlefield surgery

One of the fastest ways for a surgeon to develop his skills was to follow the advice of Hippocrates: "He who wishes to be a surgeon should go to war." Surgeons not only obtained plenty of practice on battlefields, but they had to think for themselves and improvise to solve problems. In the Middle Ages, battlefield experience had prompted some surgeons to be the first to challenge the traditional methods handed down from Galen.

In the sixteenth and seventeenth centuries, warfare was changing, forcing surgeons to solve new problems. Cannon, although first used in the fourteenth century, were now more efficient weapons. Cannonballs and musket shot were far more damaging than arrows and

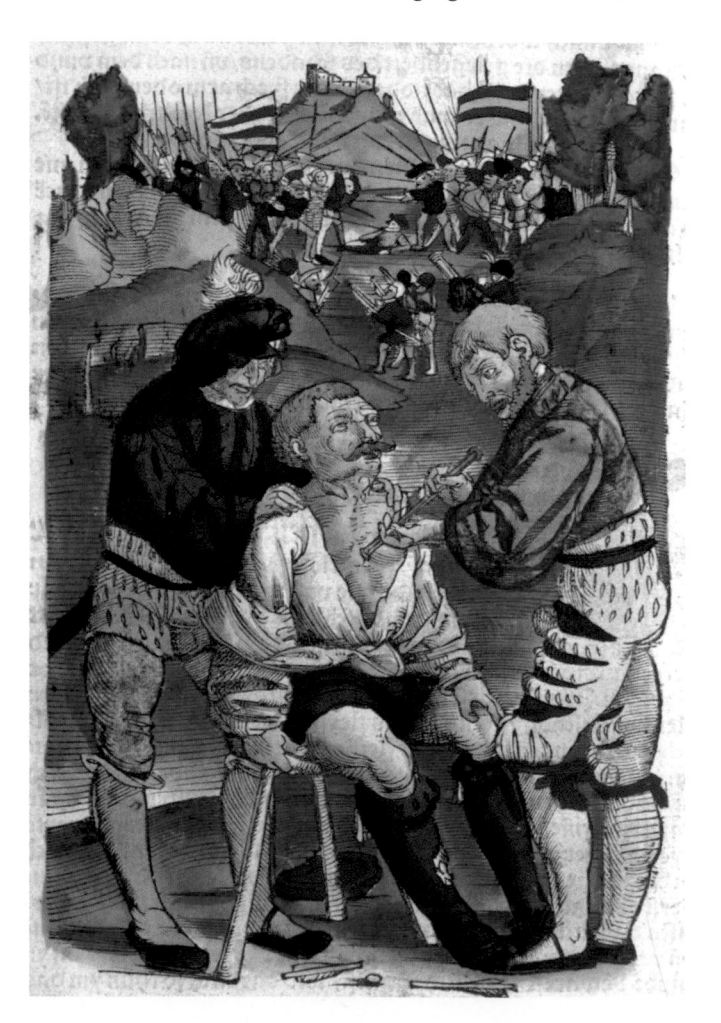

A surgeon removing an arrow from a battlefield wound, illustrated in Hans von Gersdorff's *Pocket Book of Medicine*, 1530.

swords. They tore into and destroyed a wider area of flesh and human tissue and they opened larger wounds which led to deeper and more widespread infection. People believed that gunpowder poisoned the wound, but, in reality, infection spread from fragments of clothing buried deep in the wound. To counteract infection, surgeons applied scalding hot oil or a burning iron to the wound. This did help to reduce the risk of infection in some cases, but caused agonising pain to the patient, deepening the shock from the injury.

Ambroise Paré

The battlefield and boiling oil are at the centre of the story of Ambroise Paré, the most significant surgeon of this period. Paré was born in 1510 in France and was apprenticed to his own brother who was a surgeon. After completing his training, he worked at the Hôtel Dieu in Paris, the largest hospital in France and, in 1536, became a surgeon with the French army. For the next twenty years he split his time between the army and the hospital, but it was with the army in Italy that he made his first major discovery.

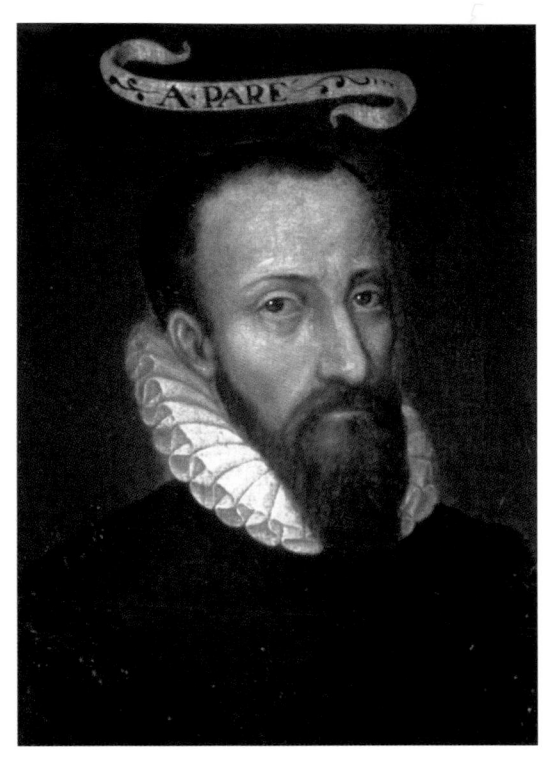

A portrait of Ambroise Paré, the French surgeon, 1510–1590.

The ideal surgeon

According to John Halle, writing in the mid-sixteenth century, a surgeon needed "a heart as the heart of a lion, his eye like the eyes of an hawk and his hands as the hands of a woman." Paré described the skills required by a good surgeon as:

... a strong, stable and intrepid hand and a resolute and merciless mind, so that he be not moved to make more haste than the thing requires, or to cut less than is needful, but does all things as if he were not affected by their cries. Nor should he give heed to the judgement of the common people, who speak ill of surgeons because of their ignorance.

Paré's chance discovery

In his book *The Apology and Treatise*, Paré described how, in 1537, he had gone against everything he had been taught about treating gunshot wounds. It was his first experience of battle and there were heavy casualties.

A surgeon cauterizing a wound. In reality the patient would not have been so placid as the burning metal touched his flesh!

"Other surgeons applied the oil, as hot as possible, into the wounds. I took courage to do as they did. Eventually I ran out of oil. I was forced instead to use an ointment made from yolks of eggs, oil of roses and turpentine. That night I could not sleep, fearing what would happen because the wounds had not been cauterized and that I should find those on whom I had not used the burning oil dead or poisoned. This made me rise up very early to visit them. To my surprise I found those to whom I gave my ointment feeling little pain, and their wounds without inflammation or swelling, having rested reasonably well during the night. The others, on whom I used the boiling oil, were feverish, with great pain and swelling around the edges of their wounds."

Leave this old and too cruel way

In *The Apology and Treatise*, published in 1585, Pare wrote:

I confess I used to staunch the bleeding after amputation in a way of which I am ashamed. I had observed my masters. They used various hot irons and caustic medicines which they would apply to the dismembered part. This thing cannot be spoken, without great horror. For this kind of remedy could not but bring great and tormenting pain to the patient. I earnestly entreat all surgeons to leave this old and too cruel way of healing and embrace this new, which was taught me by God, for I learned it not from my masters.

Chance had played its part in Paré's discovery, because he might never have tried his ointment if there had not been so many casualties and he had not run out of oil. However, his skill, knowledge and willingness to experiment were equally important. Oil and turpentine had provided some protection against infection and had not damaged the flesh as the boiling oil had done.

Paré's ligatures

Paré's belief in the importance of experiment also led him to a new method of preventing bleeding after amputations. The usual method was to press a red-hot cautery against the stump of the limb. This method sealed the blood vessels, preventing the patient bleeding to death, but the pain was excruciating. Paré's method was more time-consuming but far less painful. He tied a silk thread, called a 'ligature' around each blood vessel, which stopped the bleeding just as effectively.

An idealized picture of an amputation, with nobody needing to hold the patient down! This illustration and the one opposite are from Hans von Gersdorff's *Pocket Book of Medicine,* 1530.

Reactions to Paré's ideas

Paré became surgeon to successive French kings and published books describing his methods. He wrote in French, which could be read by more surgeons than could Latin, and his books were soon translated into other languages and read all over Europe. Earlier writers had suggested using ligatures, but Paré used his experience to explain the practical details. An English surgeon, William Clowes, reported a successful amputation at the thigh in 1588 as a result. However, there were problems. Fifty-three ligatures were needed for a thigh amputation and so a surgeon needed trained assistants, who were rare. More importantly, the ligatures themselves could carry infection into the wound, so they would not be fully effective until antiseptics were developed to kill infections.

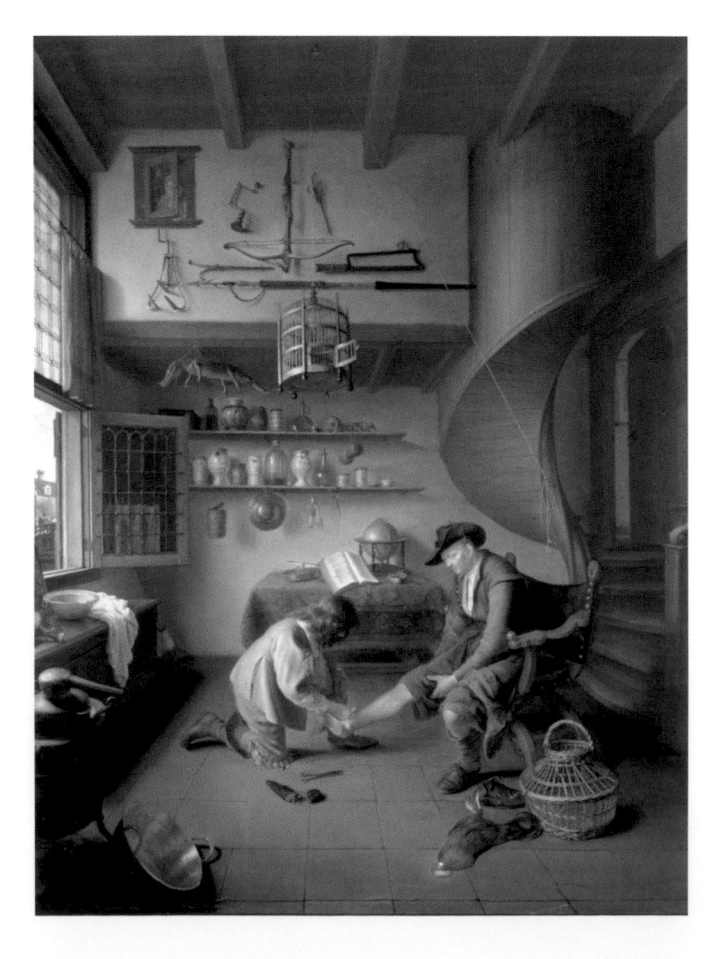

A Dutch surgeon tending a patient's foot, painted by Issac Koedyck c. 1650.

The other problem for surgeons was time. The English surgeon Richard Wiseman admired Paré's work and wrote that Paré "proposes a more easy and sure way [of closing wounds] passing the needle with a good strong thread through the skin" but advised his own readers that, in battle, there was not always time for such methods. Wiseman advised surgeons to keep "your cauteries in readiness. Use them. They will secure your patient from immediate danger".

Paré also designed false limbs for wounded soldiers, such as this artificial hand. Armourers skilled in metalworking often made the false limbs. Some artificial hands even allowed the user to grip a sword and fight.

The limits of surgery

Surgeons such as Paré and Wiseman and many others who worked humbly in towns throughout Europe did help many patients. However, the kind of operations we think of today as routine surgery – removing an appendix, for example – were still impossible to perform. They would not be possible until doctors acquired a fuller understanding of anatomy and physiology. Surgeons also needed reliable anaesthetics to replace drugs such as laudanum and henbane. Finally, operations would always be very risky until doctors understood what caused infections in wounds and then learned how to prevent infections developing. When Pepys risked that terrible operation in 1658, these developments were still 200 years away.

The reality of an amputation

An operation was not a calm event before the days of anaesthetics. The Italian doctor Fabricius described how one operation almost ended in disaster:

I was about to cut off the thigh of a man of forty years of age, and was ready to use the saw and cauteries. But the sick man began to roar out and all my assistants ran away, except only my eldest son who was then but little and to whom I had committed the holding of the patient's thigh. If my wife, then great with child, had not come running out of the next chamber and clapped hold round the patient's chest, both he and myself would have been in the greatest danger.

Chapter 6

Plague – death, suffering and prevention

For over three hundred years, bubonic plague stalked the people of Europe. Its first and greatest outbreak began in 1347, killing 20 per cent of the 100 million people of Europe and Asia. Some countries, such as Britain, suffered a death rate of over 40 per cent. From 1347 until 1722 outbreaks of plague continued in towns throughout Europe. The last major outbreak was at Marseilles in France in 1720, which killed 50,000 people – half the city's population. One of the best-recorded outbreaks of plague was the Great Plague of London, which began in 1665.

On 7 June 1665, Samuel Pepys noted in his diary: "I did in Drury Lane see two or three houses marked with a red cross upon the doors and 'Lord have mercy upon

A detail from a painting of the town hall and central square in Marseilles, at the height of the outbreak of plague that began in 1720. It is likely that this outbreak began when the city's quarantine regulations, designed to stop any sick people entering the city, failed.

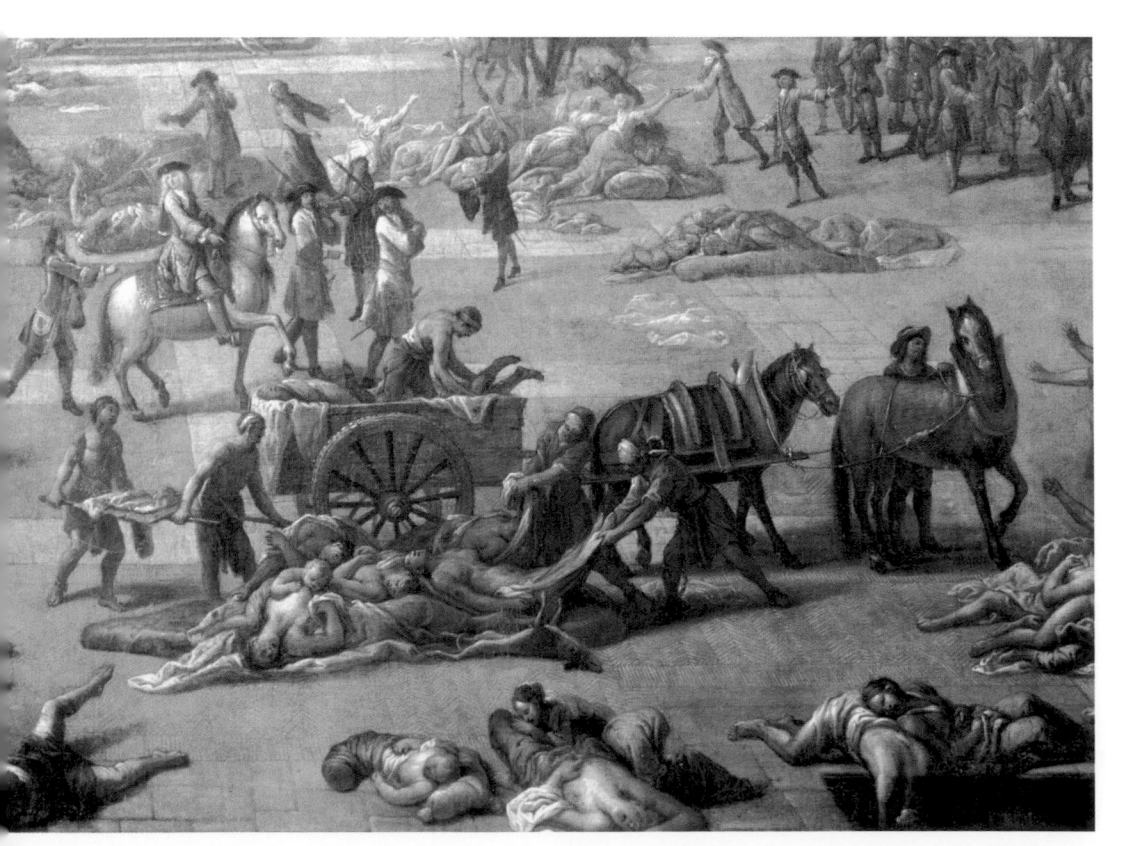

us' writ there." Thus began an outbreak of plague that over six months killed around 100,000 people – a quarter of the city's population.

A punishment from God?

The plague spread to humans from fleas that lived on the millions of rats scuttling amidst the dirt of London's streets. However, people's explanations for the epidemic were very similar to the explanations for the arrival of the Black Death 300 years earlier. Many believed that the plague had been sent by God as a punishment for their sins. Therefore the government ordered days of public prayer and fasting so that people could publicly confess their sins and beg God to be merciful and so end the plague. Fear and helplessness led others to blame the malevolent movements of the planets or poisonous air, as you can read in the panel.

This illustration shows the protective clothing worn by Italian medical examiners when they came into contact with plague victims in the seventeenth century.

Some explanations for the plague

Some ideas about the causes of plague were no different to those in the 1340s, when people blamed the arrival of the Black Death on the movements of planets. This extract is from Daniel Defoe's *Journal of the Plague Year*, published in 1722, an account of the plague based on research into documents and people's recollections:

... a blazing star or comet appeared for several months before the plague. The old women remarked that those two comets passed directly over the city ... astrologers added stories of the conjunctions of the planets. One of these conjunctions did happen in October and the other in November; and they filled the people's heads with predictions on these signs of the heavens, that they foretold drought, famine and pestilence ...

Avoiding the plague

As the plague spread, people did their best not to catch it. One of the most common beliefs was that plague was caused by 'bad air'. Therefore many people tried to fight off the smell of the 'bad air' by carrying sweet-smelling flowers, smoking tobacco or burning brimstone (sulphur) in their living rooms and workplaces. Many also wore lucky charms that they believed would ward off the plague. In his semi-fictional account, *Journal of the Plague Year*, Daniel Defoe described how:

...when anyone bought a joint of meat in the market they would not take it off the butchers' hand, but took it off the hooks themselves. On the other hand, the butcher would not touch the money, but have it put into a pot full of vinegar ... The infection generally came into the houses of citizens by means of their servants, whom they were obliged to send for food or physic [medicine] and who meet with distempered people, who conveyed the fatal breath into them.

Right: A general mortality bill for 15–22 August 1665, listing the number of deaths in each parish in London and how many of them were from the plague. This kind of evidence demonstrated how the plague hit the crowded, poorest parishes hardest.

One reason that plague spread was that people fleeing from the towns carried the disease into country villages. This illustration from a plague broadsheet shows townspeople fleeing to the country from an outbreak of plague in 1630.

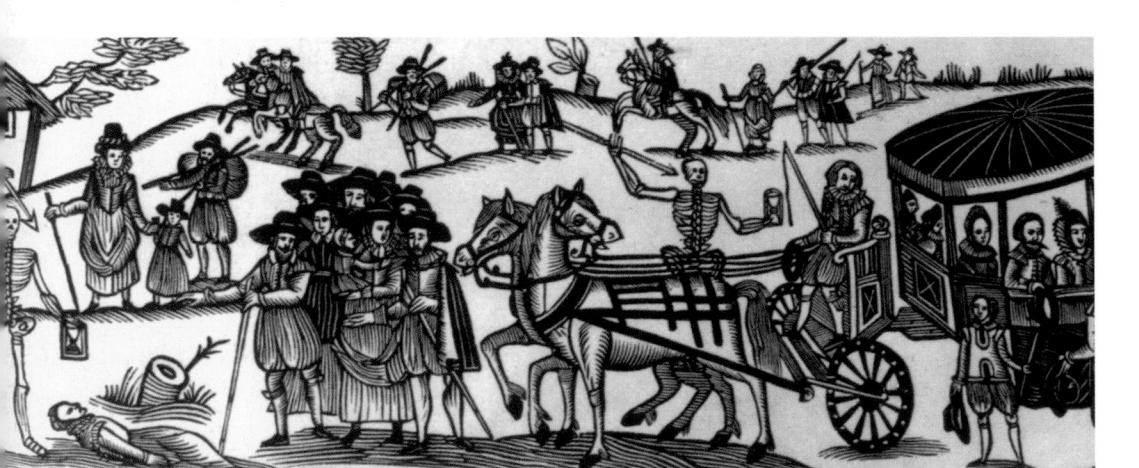

Amidst the panic, careful records were being kept, in the form of the weekly 'Bills of Mortality', listing the numbers of deaths in each parish. From these lists, some observers realized that the highest numbers of deaths were in the poorest and dirtiest parishes, where people were living crammed together in the worst housing conditions.

London 35	From the 15 of August to the 22.		1665

	Bur.	Plag.		Bur.	Plag.		Bur.	Plag.
St Alban Woodstreet-	11	8	St George Botolphlane-			St Martin Ludgate-	4	4
Alhallows Barking-	13	11	St Gregory by St Pauls-	9	5	St Martin Orgars-	8	6
Alhallows Breadstreet-	1	1	St Hellen-	11	11	St Martin Outwitch-	1	
Alhallows Great-	6	5	St James Dukes place-	7	5	St Martin Vintrey-	17	17
Alhallows Honylane-			St James Garlickhithe-	3	1	St Matthew Fridastreet-	1	
Alhallows Lesse-	3	2	St John Baptist-	7	4	St Maudlin Milkstreet-	2	2
Alhallows Lumbardstreet-	6	4	St John Evangelist-			St Maudlin Oldfishstreet-	8	4
Alhallows Stayning-	7	5	St John Zachary-	1	1	St Michael Bassishaw-	12	11
Alhallows the Wall-	23	11	St Katharine Coleman-	5	1	St Michael Cornhil-	3	1
St Alphage-	18	10	St Katharine Crechurch-	7	4	St Michael Crookedlane-	7	4
St Andrew Hubbard-	1		St Lawrence Jewry-	2	1	St Michael Queenhithe-	7	6
St Andrew Undershaft-	14	9	St Lawrence Pountney-	6	5	St Michael Quern-	1	
St Andrew Wardrobe-	21	16	St Leonard Eastcheap-	1	1	St Michael Royal-	2	1
St Ann Aldersgate-	18	11	St Leonard Fosterlane-	17	13	St Michael Woodstreet-	2	1
St Ann Blackfryers-	22	17	St Magnus Parish-	2	2	St Mildred Breadstreet-	2	1
St Antholins Parish-			St Margaret Lothbury-	2	1	St Mildred Poultrey-	4	3
St Austins Parish-			St Margaret Moses-	1		St Nicholas Acons-		
St Bartholomew Exchange	2	2	St Margaret Newfishstre.	1		St Nicholas Coleabby-	1	
St Bennet Fynch-	2	2	St Margaret Pattons-	1		St Nicholas Olaves-	3	1
St Bennet Gracechurch-			St Mary Abchurch-	1		St Olave Hartstreet-	7	4
St Bennet Paulswharf-	16	8	St Mary Aldermanbury-	11	5	St Olave Jewry-	1	1
St Bennet Sherehog-			St Mary Aldermary-	2	1	St Olave Silverstreet-	23	15
St Botolph Billingsgate-	2		St Mary le Bow-	6	6	St Pancras Soperlane-		
Christ Church-	27	22	St Mary Botham-	1	1	St Peter Cheap-	1	1
St Christophers-	1		St Mary Colechurch-			St Peter Cornhil-	7	6
St Clement Eastcheap-	2	2	St Mary Hill-	2	1	St Peter Paulswharf-	5	2
St Dionis Backchurch-	2	1	St Mary Mounthaw-	1		St Peter Poor-	3	2
St Dunstan East-	7	2	St Mary Sommerset-	6	5	St Steven Colemanstreet-	15	11
St Edmund Lumbardstr.	2	2	St Mary Stayning-	1		St Steven Walbrook-		
St Ethelborough-	13	7	St Mary Woolchurch-	1		St Swithin-	2	2
St Faith-	6	6	St Mary Woolnoth-	1	1	St Thomas Apostles-	8	7
St Foster-	13	11	St Martin Iremongerlane-			Trinity Parish-	5	3
St Gabriel Fenchurch-	1							

Christned in the 97 Parishes within the Walls —— 34   Buried —— 538   Plague —— 366

	Bur.	Plag.		Bur.	Plag.		Bur.	Plag.
St Andrew Holburn-	232	220	St Botolph Aldgate-	258	242	Saviours Southwark-	160	120
St Bartholomew Great-	58	50	St Botolph Bishopgate-	288	236	S Sepulchres Parish-	403	274
St Bartholomew Lesse-	19	15	St Dunstan West-	36	29	St Thomas Southwark-	24	21
St Bridget-	147	119	St George Southwark-	80	60	Trinity Minories-	8	5
Bridewel Precinct-	7	5	St Giles Cripplegate-	817	572	at the Pesthouse-	9	9
St Botolph Aldersgate-	70	61	St Olave Southwark-	235	131			

Christned in the 16 Parishes without the Walls—61   Buried, and at the Pesthouse—2851   Plague—2139

	Bur.	Plag.		Bur.	Plag.		Bur.	Plag.
St Giles in the fields-	204	175	Lambeth Parish-	13	9	St Mary Islington-	50	45
Hackney Parish-	12	8	St Leonard Shoreditch-	252	168	St Mary Whitechappel-	319	270
St James Clerkenwel-	172	172	St Magdalen Bermondsey	57	36	Stepney Parish-	7	5
St Kath. near the Tower	45	34	St Mary Newington-	74	52	Stepney Parish-	371	273

Christned in the 12 out Parishes in Middlesex and Surrey — 49   Buried—1571   Plague—1244

	Bur.	Plag.		Bur.	Plag.		Bur.	Plag.
St Clement Danes-	94	78	St Martin in the fields-	255	193	St Margaret Westminster	220	191
St Paul Covent Garden-	18	16	St Mary Savoy-	11	10	Whereof at the Pesthouse-		13

Christned in the 5 Parishes in the City and Liberties of Westminster—27   Buried—598   Plague—488

K 3.

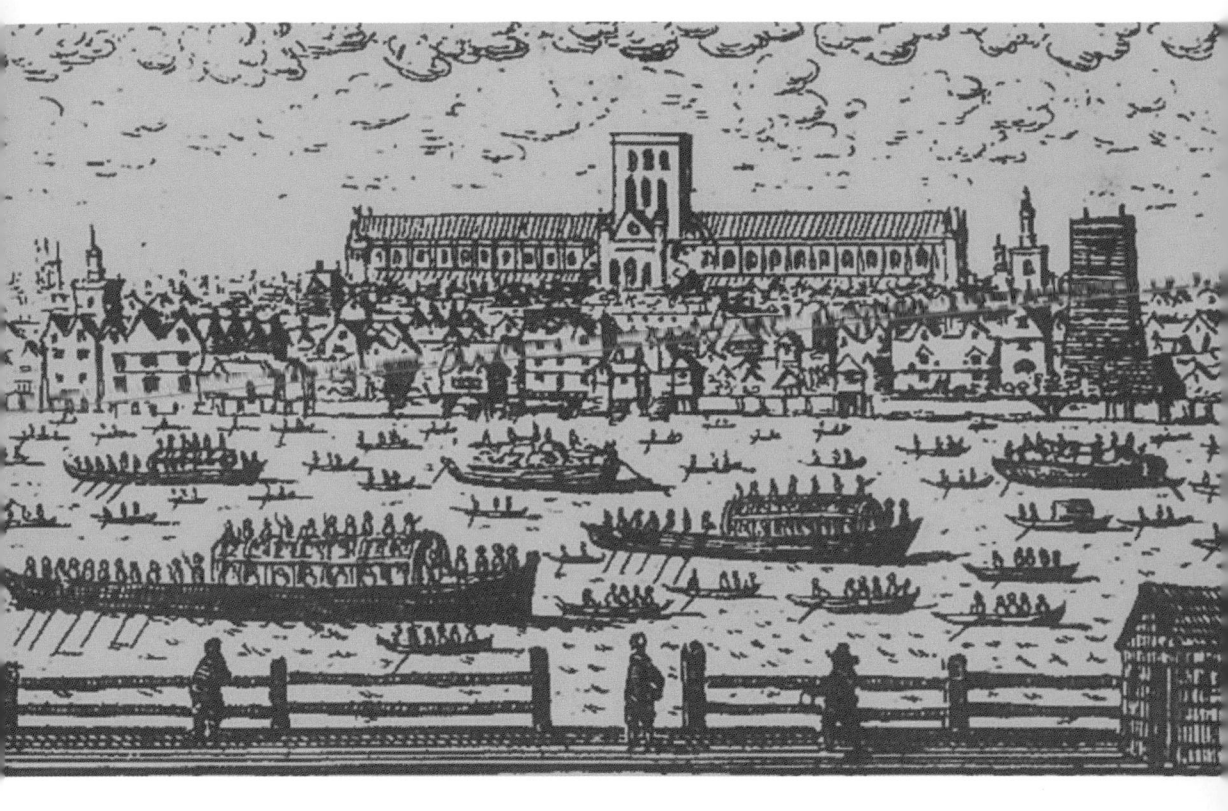

Fighting the plague

Doctors had many cures for the plague but none that
was successful. Many physicians followed their wealthy
clients into the countryside, but some stayed, including
Dr George Thomson who carried out an autopsy on a
plague victim, hoping to learn more about the disease.
Thomson caught the plague but survived, despite his
own remedy of putting a dried toad on his chest when
he felt the first symptoms.

The Mayor of London did his best to stop the plague
spreading. Ideally, victims would have been sent to
isolation hospitals, but there were only five of these and
the largest took only 90 patients, at a time when
thousands were falling ill each week. Sufferers were
shut up in their homes, the door marked with a red
cross and the words 'Lord have mercy upon us'.
Watchmen stood guard outside every infected house to
stop anyone going in or out. When anyone died, the
body was examined by 'women searchers' to check that

The River Thames was a
major transport route and
many people used the river to
escape from London at the
height of the plague.

plague was the cause and their findings were confirmed by surgeons. Bedding had to be hung in the smoke of fires before it was used again. Fires were also lit in many streets to cleanse the air of the poisons that were believed to be one of the causes of the disease.

Other regulations showed that people were making a connection between dirt and disease, even if they could not explain the link scientifically. All householders were ordered to sweep the street outside their door. Pigs, dogs, cats and other animals were not to be kept inside the city. Plays, bear-baitings and games were banned to prevent the assembly of large crowds and disorderly ale-houses and coffee-houses were closed down.

The coffin in the centre of the room provides a clear indication of the fate of many who caught the plague.

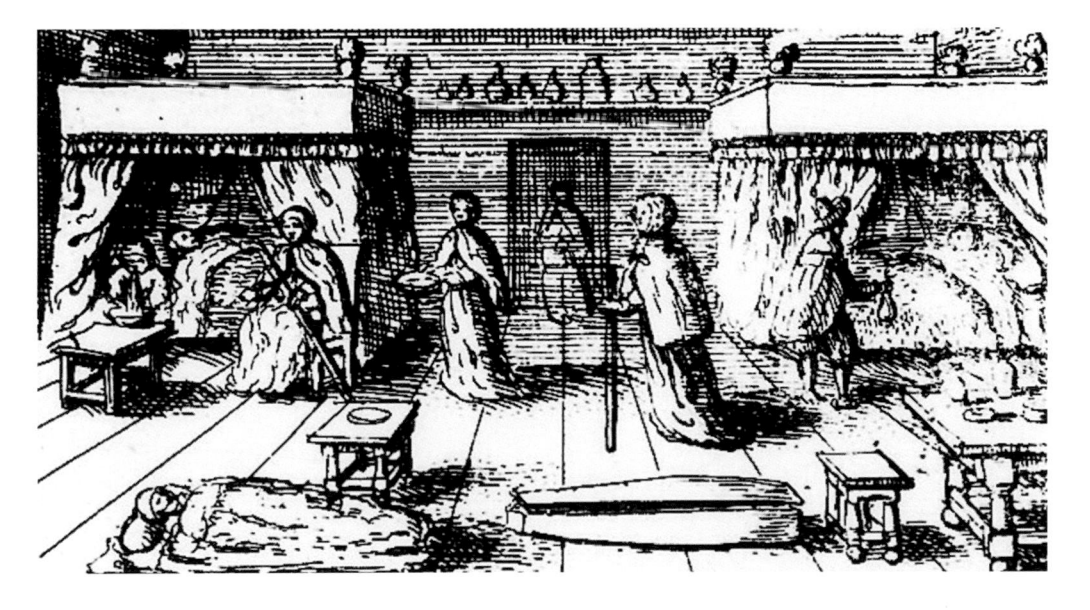

Scenes from the plague year

Thomas Vincent, a London vicar, described London during the plague:

Now shops are shut, people are rare and very few walk about, insomuch that grass begins to spring up in some places, and a deep silence in almost every place; no rattling coaches, no prancing horses, no calling in customers, nor offering wares; no London cries sounding in the ears; if any voice be heard it is the groans of dying persons, breathing forth their last, and the funeral knells of them that are ready to be carried to their graves.

Isolation hospitals

The frequent outbreaks of plague across Europe gradually changed the methods used by town and national authorities to stop it spreading. The city-states of Italy led the way. The Venetian trading colony of Ragusa (modern Dubrovnik in Croatia) was the first to keep people suspected of carrying plague in isolation, for a *trentino* – a period of 30 days. Later this was extended to *quarantenaria* – 40 days – from which the English word 'quarantine' originates. Isolation hospitals were built in Milan and Venice to keep plague victims away from the rest of the populace. While in isolation, the goods and clothes of infected people were destroyed. Boards of health checked that regulations were obeyed.

In England, where the royal government was not expected to protect people's health, there was less effective action. The government did issue some orders, such as saying that bundles of straw should be hung as a warning sign outside the homes of plague victims and that people who came from infected houses should carry a white stick in public. However, little was done to enforce regulations, partly because of the cost of employing people to enforce them at a time when there was no police force.

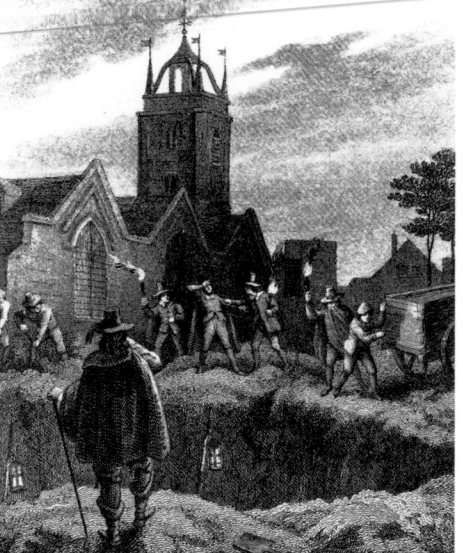

Burials took place at night so they would cause less alarm and lessen the risk of spreading plague. This illustration of *The Great Pit in Aldgate* drawn by George Cruikshank in 1835 captures the atmosphere of fear.

Unsuccessful cures for the plague

Two suggestions from the 1660s on how to help plague sufferers:

To draw the poison from the plague sore, take the feathers from the tail of a chicken and apply the chicken to the sore. The chick will gasp and labour for life. When the poison is drawn by the chicken, the patient will recover.

Wrap in woollen clothes, make the sick person sweat, which if he do, keep warm until the sores begin to rise. Then apply to the sores live pigeons cut in half or else a plaster made of yolk of an egg, honey, herb of grace and wheat flour.

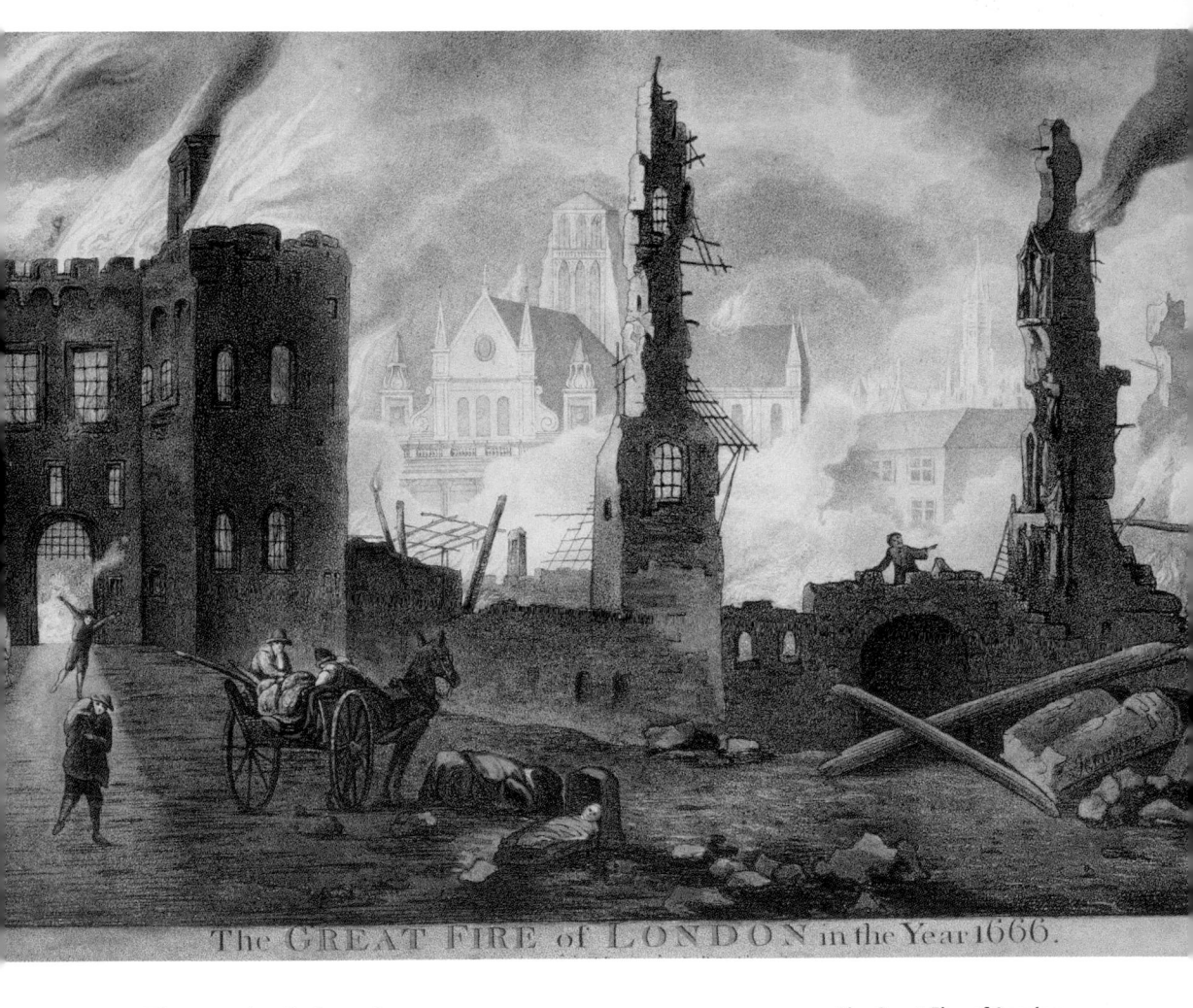

The GREAT FIRE of LONDON in the Year 1666.

The end of the plague

The cycle of plague that began in 1347 came to an end in the mid-seventeenth century, although there were occasional later outbreaks until the 1720s, such as at Marseilles (see page 48). Historians have not been able to produce a definitive explanation for the disappearance of plague, but it is likely that a number of factors played a part, including effective quarantine methods and a decline in the numbers of rats thanks to the use of an odourless, tasteless poison. Changes in the climate may also have reduced the rat population. In the seventeenth century the climate cooled, possibly changing the migration patterns of the plague-carrying rats so that far fewer came to Europe.

The Great Fire of London, which broke out in 1666, played a part in ending the cycle of plague in London by destroying many of the dirty wooden houses that had been the breeding-ground for the rats carrying the plague. This engraving is by William Birch, 1792.

Chapter 7

How successful was Renaissance medicine?

Major discoveries

The period from around 1400 to around 1750 began with the Renaissance and continued into the eighteenth century. It saw major discoveries and developments in medical science. From the time of Vesalius in the sixteenth century, doctors developed a more detailed and accurate knowledge of anatomy. There were significant breakthroughs in understanding the workings of the human body, of which the most important was Harvey's discovery that the heart pumps blood to circulate it around the body. Medical progress was aided by technological developments, such as the invention of microscopes that revealed details like the capillaries (see page 21), which previously had been invisible to the human eye.

This progress was the result of changing attitudes to knowledge. Doctors were now prepared to experiment and to challenge traditional thinking, rather than accepting ideas handed down since the Greek and Roman ages. The new emphasis on enquiry was exemplified by the development throughout Europe of societies dedicated to uncovering new scientific

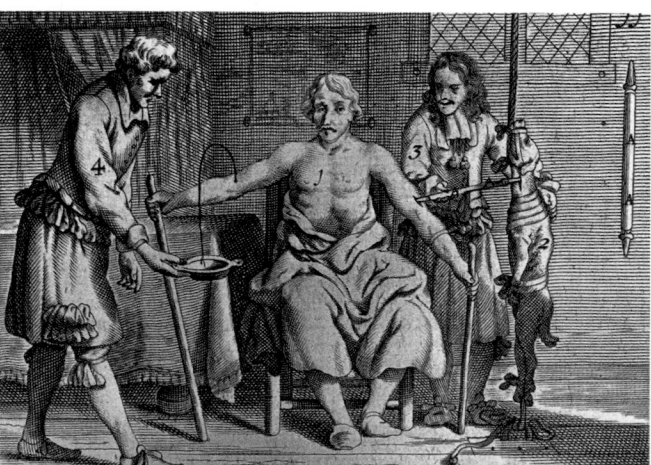

A seventeenth-century woodcut showing an attempt to transfuse blood from a dog to a man. Doctors were eager to find a way of replacing blood because accidents or operations could lead to a person bleeding to death. Some doctors experimented by getting patients to drink blood.

knowledge. In London, for example, the Royal Society organized talks and experiments by leading scientists including, at the end of the seventeenth century, some of the earliest experiments in blood transfusions, from dog to dog, then from dog to human and finally from human to human. There were occasional successes, but transfusion could not be a regular success until scientists identified the people's different blood groups.

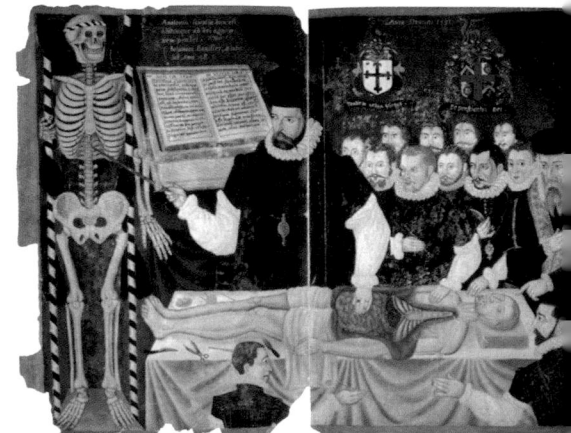

John Bannister delivering an anatomy lesson in a late sixteenth-century or early seventeenth-century painting.

Raising expectations

Discoveries also raised expectations. When Samuel Pepys feared he was going blind, he was alarmed to discover that Dr Turberville, the leading expert on eye problems, had only once witnessed an eye being dissected.

This period therefore laid the basis for the revolution in medicine that took place after 1800. However, the advances in medical science had little impact on people's health. As the writer John Aubrey noted in 1680, "All his profession agree Dr Harvey to be an excellent anatomist, but I never heard any that admired his treatment of the sick. I knew several doctors in London that would not have given threepence for one of his prescriptions." As the panel shows, even the most everyday medical treatments could still be an agonising and fearful experience.

Drawing a tooth

This extract is from James Woodforde's diary 4 June, 1776:

My tooth pained me all night, got up a little after 5 and sent for Reeves, a man who draws teeth and about 7 he came and drew my tooth, but shockingly bad indeed, he broke away a great piece of my gum and broke one of the fangs of the tooth. It gave me exquisite pain all the day after and my face was swelled prodigiously in the evening and much pain. Paid the old man that drew it however. He is too old, I think, to draw teeth, can't see very well.

Life expectancy

People did not live longer as a result of the scientific discoveries of this period. The number of deaths in childhood was still very high, as babies and children were extremely vulnerable to infections. There was also a high death rate amongst women in childbirth. The result was that less than half the population of Europe lived to the age of 40.

There were also periods, in all countries, when the death rate increased significantly because poor harvests led to a badly nourished population who were more vulnerable to disease. In the 1550s in England "the scarcity of bread was so great that the poor people did eat acorns and a sickness of strong fever did sore molest them." Around twenty per cent of the English population died at that time from famine and influenza. This danger continued in Britain until the late eighteenth century when the agricultural revolution increased the amounts of food grown and food also began to be imported in large quantities. In other countries, such as Russia, which were slower to change their agricultural methods, the danger of famine continued into the early twentieth century.

This graph shows the age at death of 250 people from the parish of Adel in Yorkshire between 1685 and 1700. The figures on the bars total 250.

Life expectancy in the 1600s

The history of Samuel Pepys' family tells us that people were not living any longer in the 1600s than they had done in the Middle Ages or any earlier period of history. Pepys himself lived to be 70 and his parents also lived to a good age, his father living to be 79 and his mother 60. However, of Samuel's ten brothers and sisters, six died before the age of 10, one died at 13 and only three reached adulthood, all dying between the ages of 30 and 40. The Pepys family is very typical of this period. A few people lived a long life, but the majority died young.

The major reason for so many early deaths was that doctors still did not understand exactly why people became ill and therefore could not develop effective cures or methods of preventing disease. However, the pace of medical change was increasing. By the mid-eighteenth century, medical beliefs that had held sway since the Greek and Roman periods were being discarded. A foundation of knowledge was being established that would provide the launch pad for the revolution in medicine and health that took place in the nineteenth and twentieth centuries. Ahead lay Louis Pasteur's discovery of bacteria and their role in disease, together with the public health reforms that would win the battle against the dirt that helped breed disease. This medical revolution was built on the foundations laid between the years 1450 and 1750.

Louis Pasteur (1822–1896) was the French scientist who developed the germ theory, which suggested that bacteria are the true cause of disease. Pasteur's careful scientific methods, based on experiment and observation, owed a great deal to the methods developed by Renaissance scientists.

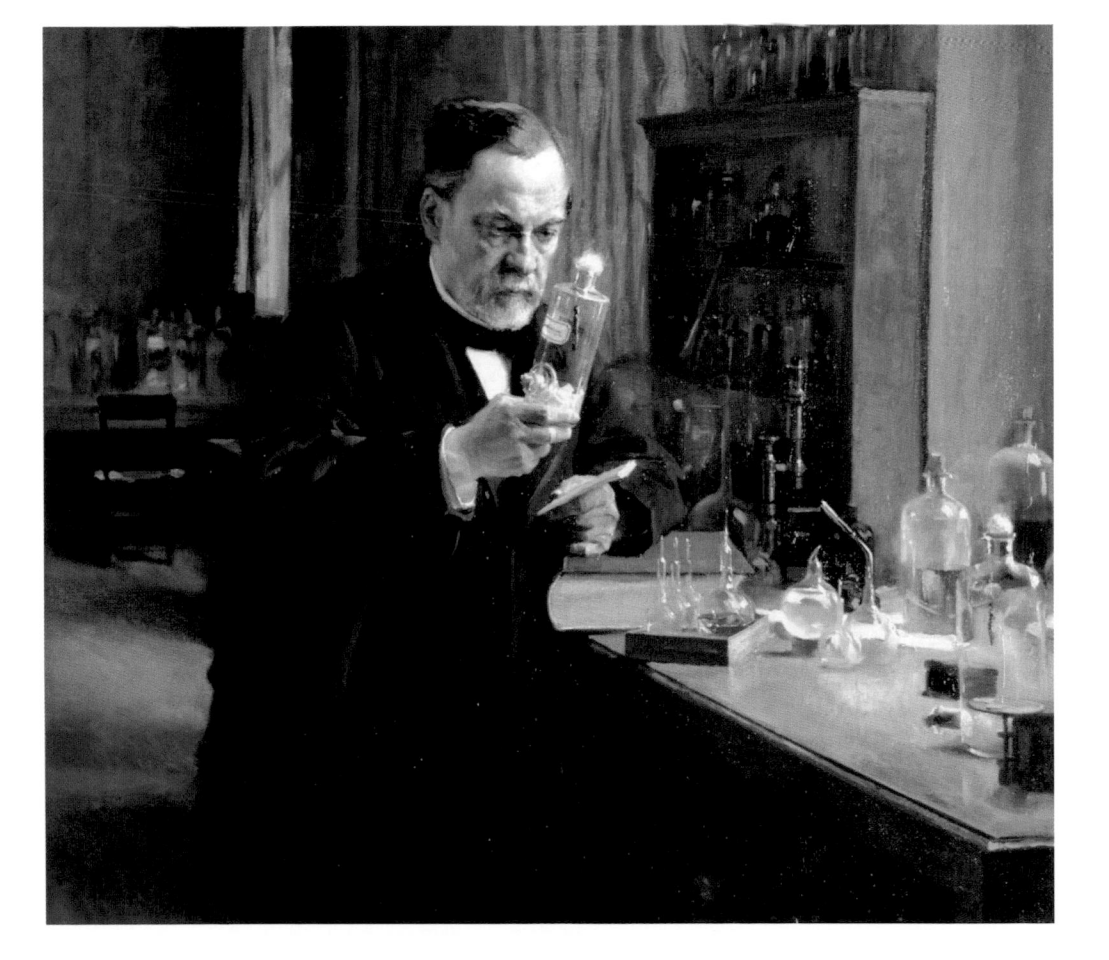

Anaemia a condition caused by a lack of iron in the blood

Anaesthetic a drug that induces pain relief, used mainly in preparation for surgery, sometimes making the person unconscious

Anatomy the study of the structure of the human body

Antidote a medicine that counteracts a poison

Antiseptic a chemical or a natural substance that destroys bacteria and kills infection

Apothecary a pharmacist or chemist

Arteries the blood vessels that carry blood away from the heart

Astrology the study of the planets and how they might influence people's lives

Astronomy the study of the stars and planets

Barber-surgeon a barber who often combined this role with performing minor surgery, e.g. lancing boils etc.

Capillaries the invisible vessels in the human body that transfer blood from the arteries to the veins

Cartilage gristle or tissue that forms part of the joints of the body

Cautery a hot piece of iron used to burn the flesh around an open wound; this process helps to seal the wound and so stop bleeding

Chilblains swellings on the toes or fingers caused by constriction of the blood vessels in cold weather

Colic severe, occasional pain

Dismembered cut off or separated limb from limb

Distempered suffering from sickness

Dissection the cutting up and scientific examination of the human body

Dysentery a severe illness causing frequent, fluid bowel movements

Efficacious efficient and helpful

Epidemic a disease affecting a large number of people at once

Expectorant a medicine used to make the patient cough up phlegm

Famine a severe shortage of food leading to starvation

Femur the thigh bone

Gibbet the gallows where people were hanged

Henbane a poisonous plant and the drug obtained from the plant, sometimes used as an anaesthetic

Immunity protection against a disease

Inoculate to infect someone with a slight dose of a disease in order to develop immunity for the future

Jaundice an illness of the liver, whose most obvious symptom is yellowing of the face

Laudanum a drug, based on opium, used as a painkiller

Ligature a thread tied around a blood vessel to stop bleeding

Lithotomy an operation to remove stones from the bladder

Membrane a thin lining or covering of an organ or other part of the body

Midwife a woman who assists at a birth

Musket an early form of rifle

Obstetrics the study of childbirth and midwifery

Opium a drug obtained from the poppy plant; it makes people sleepy and was used as an anaesthetic

Pharmacist someone who studies and makes drugs for use as medicines

Physician a university-trained doctor

Physiology the study of how the body works

Purge to cleanse the body by taking drugs that make people vomit or empty their bowels

Quacks healers with no professional training

Scarlet fever an infectious disease, common in childhood

Scurvy a disease caused by not taking in enough vitamin C, which is found mostly in fruit and vegetables; scurvy causes blood loss which can eventually affect the brain and cause death

Septum a membrane in the middle of the heart

Sinews a tendon that joins a muscle to a bone

Smallpox a disease that is similar to influenza; it leads to a severe rash and blisters; it has affected humans for many centuries but became much more dangerous from the eighteenth century onwards, killing 40 per cent of sufferers

Tendons strong chords that join muscles to bone or to other muscles

Trepanning (also trephining) drilling a hole into the skull in order to relieve pressure on the brain

Tumour a swelling caused by cells reproducing at an abnormal rate

Typhoid an infectious disease, caught from contaminated food or water

Veins the blood vessels that carry blood towards the heart

Vivisection dissection of live bodies

Woodcut an illustration made by engraving the picture into a block of wood and then using the woodblock in the printing process

Events	Dates CE	People
c. 1450 The invention of the printing press by Gutenberg	**1450**	**1452** Birth of Leonardo da Vinci
1492 Columbus began the colonization of the Americas		**1493** Birth of Paracelsus, who attacked Galen's work and promoted new ideas about treatments
	1500	
1518–1531 Destruction of Aztec and Incan civilizations by smallpox carried to the Americas by Europeans		**1537** Pare developed a new method of treating gunpowder wounds
		1543 Vesalius published *The Fabric of the Human Body*
Late 1500s Chamberlen family secretly developed the obstetric forceps		
	1600	
1620s The Italian scientist Galileo developed the microscope		**1628** William Harvey published *An Anatomical Account of the Motion of the Heart and Blood in Animals*
1660s Development of more effective microscopes by Malphigi, Hooke and van Leeuwenhoek		
1665 Outbreak of plague in London		
	1700	
1720 Marseilles suffered the last outbreak in the plague cycle, which had begun in 1348		**1720** Lady Mary Wortley Montagu brought the idea of inoculation from Turkey to Britain

Books

Blood and Guts, A Short History of Medicine,
Roy Porter, Penguin, 2002

The Illustrated History of Surgery,
Knut Haeger, Harold Starke, 2000
An entertaining, up-to-date history for older readers.

Health and Medicine through Time,
Ian Dawson and Ian Coulson, John Murray, 1996
The most widely used schoolbook for examinations on this topic.

The Terrible Tudors,
Terry Deary, Scholastic Hippo, 1993

The Slimy Stuarts,
Terry Deary, Scholastic Hippo, 1996
Entertaining, funny and informative.

The Young Oxford History of Britain and Ireland,
Kenneth O. Morgan (editor), Oxford University Press, 1996

History Detective Investigates Tudor Medicine,
Richard Tames, Hodder Wayland, 2002

You Wouldn't Want to Be Ill in Tudor Times,
Kathryn Senior, Hodder Wayland, 2002

Renaissance,
Andrew Langley, Eyewitness series, Random House Children's Books, 1999

Renaissance,
Alison Cole, Dorling Kindersley, 2000
A selection of well-illustrated information books on daily life and other key aspects of Renaissance and early modern history.

Websites

www.renaissance.dm.net
A guide to daily life during the Renaissance with links to other sites dealing with the period.

www.medhist.ac.uk
A guide to websites on the history of medicine, chiefly aimed at an academic audience.

www.spartacus.schoolnet.co.uk
A wide-ranging site that includes links to many sites covering ancient history.

www.english-heritage.org.uk
Information on castles, stately homes and other sites from this period in Britain that are open to the public.

www.thebritishmuseum.ac.uk
Details and visuals of the museum's collections, which include objects from the period 1450–1750.

www.medicalmuseums.org
A guide to ten medical museums in and around London.

www.bl.uk/collections/treasures.html
An introduction to some of the most famous documents in the British Library's collection, including da Vinci's *Notebook* and Gutenberg's Bible.

www.nga.gov/collection
Highly-illustrated site of the National Gallery of Art, Washington DC, containing, amongst others, tours of Renaissance galleries.

www.nationalgallery.org.uk
The online guide to the collections of the National Gallery in London, including the art and artists of the Renaissance.

www.bbc.co.uk
Entertaining information on the Tudor and Stuart periods in Britain, the European Renaissance and medical and scientific topics and individuals, such as da Vinci.

www.luminarium.org
A guide to the literature of the period 1450–1650 with a large collection of links to other aspects of this period.

www.thinkinghistory.co.uk
A guide to active teaching and learning methods for schools, including examples on the history of medicine.

Places to visit

Thackray Medical Museum, Beckett Street, Leeds
Interactive displays on the history of medicine, designed for all ages.
www.thackraymuseum.org.uk

The Science Museum, London
Displays on many aspects of science, including medicine.
www.sciencemuseum.org.uk

The Museum of London
Well-presented, interactive displays on Tudor and Stuart London.
www.museumoflondon.org.uk

Index